# SURGICAL PRACTICE
# ILLUSTRATED

*David B. Skinner, Series Editor*

# ATLAS OF ESOPHAGEAL SURGERY

*David B. Skinner, M.D.*

President and Chief Executive Officer
The New York Hospital
Professor, Department of Surgery
Cornell University Medical College
New York, New York

*Illustrated by Kathy Hirsh*

**CHURCHILL LIVINGSTONE**
New York, Edinburgh, London, Melbourne, Tokyo

**Library of Congress Cataloging-in-Publication Data**

Skinner, David B., date
   Atlas of esophageal surgery / David B. Skinner ; illustrated by
Kathy Hirsh.
      p.   cm. – (Surgical practice illustrated)
   Includes index.
   ISBN 0-443-08610-9
   1. Esophagus–Surgery–Atlases.   I. Title.   II. Series
      [DNLM: 1. Esophageal Diseases–surgery–atlases.   2. Esophagus-
   -surgery–atlases.   WI 17 S628a]
   RD539.5.S58   1991
   617.5'45059–dc20
   DNLM/DLC
   for Library of Congress                         90–15184
                                                          CIP

Distributed in the United Kingdom by Churchill Livingstone, Robert Stevenson
House, 1–3 Baxter's Place, Leith Walk, Edinburgh EH1 3AF, and by associated
companies, branches, and representatives throughout the world.

Accurate indications, adverse reactions, and dosage schedules for drugs are
provided in this book, but it is possible that they may change. The reader is urged
to review the package information data of the manufacturers of the medications
mentioned.

Acquisitions Editor: *Avé McCracken*
Copy Editor: *Christina Joslin*
Book Designer: *Gloria Brown*
Production Supervisor: *Sharon Tuder*

Printed in the United States of America

First published in 1991      7 6 5 4 3 2 1

# Introduction to the Series

Although I originally turned down the prospective North American editorship of an international surgical multispecialty atlas series several years ago, I subsequently thought a lot about the merits of surgical atlases. Given the right circumstances to create an optimal series, the concept is very attractive. The conditions that create the setting and need include the recognition of the rapidly changing nature of surgery, the impact of these changes on formal surgical education, and technical developments to advance the quality of such atlases. When Churchill Livingstone proposed that the time was right for a new atlas series, I agreed with enthusiasm.

Changes in the practice and techniques of surgery in the last 25 years have been phenomenal. Inspecting operating lists for several days in major surgical centers quickly established that about 90 percent of the operations done in 1988 were either unknown or could not be done safely when I was in mid-residency in 1963. The rapid introduction of so much new knowledge has inevitably led to fragmentation and specialization. In 1963 at the Massachusetts General Hospital, the general surgery chief residency included independent operating experience in cardiac, colorectal, gynecologic, pediatric, plastic, thoracic, and vascular surgery. Today, each has its own formal specialty certification and residency review process. Included within regular general surgery training were endocrine, fracture, gastrointestinal, hand, hepatobiliary, intensive care, oncology, pancreatic, transplantation, and trauma surgery. Each of these is now offered as specialty fellowships in some hospitals and is evolving toward formal specialty recognition. Neurosurgery, orthopaedics, otolaryngology, and urology were already separate residency programs, but rotation at the junior level exposed the general surgery resident to the principles of each. The breadth of exposure to the techniques and precepts evolving in multiple specialties equipped the resident of that era with a versatility that could be applied to the more rapid evolution of the subspecialty in which he (women were almost nonexistent in surgical residencies 25 years ago) was interested. However, today, no surgeon trained in that era practices the full range of surgery that he learned in residency.

Specialization has become inevitable, and the strong forces driving it continue. The rapid growth in fundamental biomedical knowledge and its application to clinical medicine make it impossible to keep up with new advances in several disciplines. Public interest and knowledge about advances in medicine and surgery have led to a common expectation of specialized expertise. This trend has been reinforced by the credentialing procedure of leading hospitals and the risk of malpractice litigation when difficult problems are taken on by the nonspecialist no matter how able. The rapid emergence in specialization in internal medicine and nonsurgical disciplines led to referral patterns rewarding to the counterpart surgical specialist. Medical school appointments and promotions depend largely on scientific and scholarly contributions which almost by definition require focus and specialization. Finally, modern transportation is such that it is unlikely that a patient with an unusual or complicated problem is more than two hours away from a knowledgeable specialist in that problem.

On the other hand there continue to be factors encouraging more general knowledge and practice in surgery. Specialization carried to extremes is very costly to society. The total cost of medical care in the United States has reached the point where powerful forces are demanding restraint and reversal. This movement places more value on the surgeon who has breadth in his or her armamentarium. For example, HMOs, introduced as a vehicle to contain medical costs, cannot afford to employ full-time specialists in every surgical discipline, yet they have strong economic disincentives to refer out surgery on a fee for service basis. The result is that a true generalist in surgery is highly desirable and busy in an HMO practice setting. Also many procedures which were initially difficult have now become routine, safe, and readily practiced by a generalist.

As operations in the newer disciplines become standardized, they can be done as well and safely in a local setting as in the referral center. A significant portion of the public will choose the local hospital and is encouraged to do so by the local physician who will remain involved in the case. Yet, as pointed out above, these smaller population bases cannot support the full range of subspecialists; therefore, surgeons practicing in the community hospitals should remain up-to-date in several fields and add that which is becoming standardized and routine in related specialties to their own scope of practice.

The explosion in medical and surgical knowledge has extended the benefits of surgical correction to many disorders which are not life-threatening, but which interfere with function and enjoyment of life. When life or limb are at stake, higher risks are acceptable, and the surgical procedure is done with available resources and talents. However, an operation for reconstructive surgery or prophylaxis against future illness, must have minimal risks, and the functional success of the operation must be carefully evaluated. This places renewed emphasis on the details of technical surgery and assessment of its impact on the operative results. In recent times, new information on the body's responses to trauma and stress has encouraged emphasis in residency programs in intensive care practice, resuscitation, and the understanding of biochemistry, pharmacology, immunology, nutrition, and sepsis. Yet, at the same time, the evolution of surgical specialties is based substantially on technical innovations and understanding of the effect of these on tissue healing and function.

What has all this to do with the assertion that the setting and time are right for a new surgical atlas series? A medical textbook, and especially a surgical atlas, is essentially an educational tool. The assertion of need must be based on educational grounds. All of the above described changes occurring in surgery have impacted directly on both residency and continuing surgical education. The rapid and recent growth in surgical knowledge and technique means that most active surgical practitioners do not have personal experience and instruction in a number of newer valuable techniques which are being well established. The inevitable conservatism and tradition of residency programs and faculty often means that new techniques developed and taught elsewhere are not rapidly and uniformly evaluated and introduced into a particular program. The number of specialties evolving makes it unlikely that any one medical center and surgical residency can afford or indeed has up-to-date leadership in each discipline.

The value of cross-fertilization of ideas and techniques across disciplines is well appreciated, but difficult to achieve as barriers are erected among the specialties. With much emphasis appropriately placed in surgical residencies on the scientific basis and acquisition of knowledge in treating shock, infection, and immunologic and nutritional disorders, there is an understandable tendency in some programs to divert attention from or downplay the importance of technique. Yet much of the critical outcome of the newer surgery for non-life-threatening conditions depends directly on surgical technique. An optimally presented multispecialty surgical atlas series can help to address each of these concerns in the surgical residency experience and to support the surgeon desiring to acquire surgical knowledges and techniques in his practice after completion of residency.

Ideally, a surgical atlas series should offer a general education in surgery. Each component of the series should be taught by a world authority in that specialty who has personal experiences and judgment to know the variety of techniques available and to select the one most appropriate for the condition at hand and most likely to give the best technical result. In this series, the authors of each volume are surgeons personally known to me as well as generally acknowledged to be technical masters and world authorities in their specialty. Each has significant, scientific contributions to the establishment and advancement of the specialty. Each has published extensively—describing the indications, rationale, and long-term follow-up results of the techniques illustrated. The reader can easily confirm the applicability and validity of the operations described in the published literature and have confidence in its value in his or her practice. As a result, the text of the atlas can be brief, highly technical, and of the utmost practical value to the surgical resident or practitioner who seriously wishes to add excellent techniques to his or her practice base.

In parallel with the developments in surgery, surgical illustration has developed considerably in recent years and is now a more precise discipline. Although artistically gifted surgeons have illustrated their publications for centuries, formal surgical illustration is a more recent event. Max Brodel is generally acclaimed as the founder of the field of medical illustration and established the first school at Johns Hopkins University School of Medicine in 1913. Several other schools became prominent between the first and second world wars. The field acquired greater breadth, sophistication, and rapid growth after the second world war. Today artists are available to do a surgical atlas series soundly based upon detailed anatomic knowledge and personal observation of techniques in the operating room. For this series, a few such highly qualified surgical illustrators have been selected so that a high standard, based both upon artistic excellence and detailed anatomic and surgical knowledge, can be maintained throughout the series.

The changing nature of surgical practices and education, the willingness of world class operating surgeons to participate, the availability of excellent scientifically ground surgical illustrators, plus the willingness of the publishers to provide a budget to support a top quality surgical atlas series have proved irresistible to me. I hope the product will prove immensely useful to many colleagues in all surgical disciplines who stand to learn and benefit greatly from the techniques that world authorities in related surgical fields have to offer.

*David B. Skinner, M.D.*
*President and Chief Executive Officer*
*The New York Hospital*
*Professor, Department of Surgery*
*Cornell University Medical College*
*New York, New York*

# *Foreword*

Illustration is an essential element in any monograph on surgical technique. Photography is rarely informative and videos may show the surgeon attempting certain maneuvers without clearly defining their anatomic background. Maneuvers such as exposure and mobilization, which are tedious and time-consuming but equally essential, are usually deleted in videos.

Illustrations in monochrome or color follow a variety of tradition. From Leonardo da Vinci up to the time of World War II anatomic and surgical illustration was regarded as an art form and appreciated as such, rather than for any practical information on technique of possible value to the operating surgeon. Many schools for medical artists in the United States and elsewhere in the world perpetuated the tradition.

Following World War II the situation changed. The traditional "artistic" approach became too time-consuming and expensive in the face of greater demand and rapidly expanding publication. The financial rewards failed to lure competent graduates from art schools away from the more lucrative fields of commercial and fashion illustration. There arose a demand for a more economical style of illustration, not only slicker in execution but more informative in the essentials of surgical technique. Contemporary illustration can be classified into three styles: (1) the simple line diagram so successfully exploited by Lee McGregor in his prewar *Synopsis of Surgical Anatomy*; (2) the cartoon, a sketch exaggerating only the essential details of the procedure and departing from the photographic approach; and (3) a survival of the traditional "artistic" approach.

Probably the ideal style is a cartoon with only sufficient chiaroscuro to emphasize the three-dimensional anatomic relationship of the structures involved. The initial cartoon should be prepared by the operating surgeon, the one person who knows just which steps in the procedure should be emphasized, and how. The surgeon is concerned about allowing for variations in human anatomy and illustrating the average situation, with additional marginal remarks illustrating the common variants. Unfortunately few surgeons have had any training in drawing. Nevertheless they should acquire the ability to produce relevant cartoons to be handed over later to the medical artist to prepare for publication. Though it may be time-consuming, communication between surgeon and artist is essential. The artist present in the operating room observes in a photographic idiom and thus must collaborate with the surgeon, who knows how the situation should actually appear. Together, the surgeon and the artist may discard numerous preliminary drawings before final satisfaction is achieved.

I have had the pleasure of collaborating personally with the artist of this text, Kathy Hirsh. Ms. Hirsh has been involved with many projects, is intimately acquainted with the regional anatomy, and has conveyed with admirable clarity what the surgeon is demonstrating. Her technique approaches closely the ideal previously discussed. The addition of simple line drawings alongside the cartoons contributes significantly to the information. The monograph under review is unique in several respects. The author has vast practical experience in a highly specialized field and is universally recognized as a leader in this discipline. All the techniques illustrated have stood the test of time and proved their long-term value in the follow-up clinic. Having been involved personally in esophageal surgery for the last 45 years, I can appreciate the potential and unique contribution now available to other surgeons involved in this technically demanding discipline. A vast amount of essential and practical information is presented. Technical steps with which the average surgeon is already familiar have been eliminated in order to highlight the essential information acquired only by long practical experience in the field. The text is highly important and must be studied as carefully as the illustrations.

I confidently recommend this Atlas of esophageal surgical technique not only to the surgeon developing an interest in the discipline, but equally to every surgeon already involved and aware of the technical hazards that determine success or failure, early and late.

*Ronald Belsey, M.S., F.R.C.S., F.R.C.S.I. (Hon.)*
*Emeritus Professor of Cardio-Thoracic Surgery*
*Southwest Regional Cardio-Thoracic Surgery Unit*
*Bristol, England*

# *Preface*

Over the past several decades much has been learned about esophageal disorders, and surgical techniques have been developed to correct or palliate related diseases not previously treated. It was my good fortune during the years 1962 to 1964 to be introduced to esophageal surgery under the guidance of two acknowledged masters who developed the field. As a resident at Massachusetts General Hospital, I served with Dr. Richard Sweet who was regarded worldwide as a preeminent esophageal surgeon from World War II until his retirement in 1962. The complexity and challenge of esophageal disorders stimulated my lifelong interest. Shortly thereafter, Professor Edward Churchill made arrangements for me to serve as Senior Registrar for Mr. Ronald Belsey at the Frenchay Hospital in Bristol, England. I learned Mr. Belsey's highly innovative, simplified, and elegant approach to esophageal disease and its surgical treatment.

Ronald Belsey developed a number of new techniques, several of which are illustrated in this Atlas including the world famous Mark IV antireflux repair; cricopharyngeal myotomy and diverticulopexy simplifying the treatment of Zenker's diverticulum; modification of the Heller myotomy to include an antireflux repair; standardization of the isoperistaltic left colon interposition for esophageal replacement; and the exclusive right thoracotomy approach to esophagectomy and advancement of the stomach through the hiatus for reconstruction. Of even greater importance to me, Ronald and I developed a lifelong collaboration and friendship persisting to this day, and resulting in our recent book, *Management of Esophageal Disease*, which describes in detail the indications, investigations, and rationale for, and the experience resulting from the operations illustrated in this Atlas.

Upon returning to the Massachusetts General Hospital, I was motivated by the Bristol experience to develop and put into practice esophageal function tests based on intra-esophageal pH recordings and the application of en bloc principles for treating carcinoma of the intrathoracic esophagus. In subsequent years on the faculty at the School of Aerospace Medicine and Wilfred Hall U.S.A.F. Hospital in San Antonio, Texas, at Johns Hopkins Hospital, at the University of Chicago Pritzker School of Medicine, and now at The New York Hospital-Cornell Medical Center, I have been fortunate to have a series of outstanding fellows, residents, and colleagues who have collaborated in studies of esophageal diseases and treatment, and whose contributions to the field have been enormous.

Based on more than 25 years of investigation, extensive operative experience, and follow-up of patients with esophageal disease, the techniques in this Atlas are presented as used and taught in my current practice. The key to successful esophageal surgery is correct preoperative investigations and diagnosis. Many of the failures of surgical treatment result from inappropriate application of various operations depicted. The reader of this Atlas is strongly urged to learn and apply the methods for precise preoperative analysis of patients with esophageal disorders and indications for the various operations. Ongoing long-term follow-up is essential to assess the effectiveness of the surgical treatments.

The illustrations have been done by Kathy Hirsh, a longtime collaborator and friend. Kathy has spent hours in the operating room observing the procedures that she has illustrated. She has revised the drawings a number of times to make them as accurate and realistic as possible. This is the second volume that Ms. Hirsh has illustrated in the *Surgical Practice Illustrated* Series, the first being the *Atlas of Vascular Surgery* by Christopher K. Zarins and Bruce L. Gewertz. Her illustrations in the first volume are widely acclaimed, and she has done an equally superb job in illustrating these complicated esophageal procedures.

*David B. Skinner, M.D.*

# Contents

**I**    *Operative Approaches to the Esophagus*    **1**

    1   Abdominal Approaches    2

    2   Thoracic Approach—Left Thoracotomy    6

    3   Thoracic Approach—Right Thoracotomy    10

    4   Approaches to the Cervical Esophagus    12

    5   Cervical Approach Combined With Partial Sternotomy    16

**II**    *Resection for Malignant Neoplasms*    **19**

    1   En Bloc Esophagectomy Through a Left Thoracotomy    20

    2   En Bloc Esophagectomy Through a Right Thoracotomy    32

    3   Standard or Palliative Esophagectomy Through a Right Thoracotomy    36

    4   Esophagectomy Without Thoracotomy    42

**III**    *Reconstructions of the Esophagus*    **53**

    1   Reconstruction With the Whole Stomach    54

    2   Reconstruction With Isoperistaltic Left Colon    62

    3   Long Segment Interposition    72

    4   Anastomotic Techniques    76

    5   Continuous Suture Anastomotic Technique    78

    6   Jejunal Interposition    80

    7   Gastric Tube Interposition    90

    8   Reconstructions After Total Gastrectomy: Jejunal Loop    92

    9   Reconstructions After Total Gastrectomy: Isoperistaltic Left Colon    96

**IV**    *Bypass Procedures*    **99**

    1   Substernal Left Colon Bypass    100

    2   Substernal Stomach Bypass    108

    3   Subcutaneous Right Colon Bypass    110

**V** | *Antireflux Repairs* **115**

    1   Transthoracic Antireflux Repairs: Belsey Mark IV Operation    116

    2   Transthoracic Nissen Fundoplication    124

    3   Transabdominal Antireflux Repairs: Nissen Fundoplication    128

    4   The Hill Posterior Gastropexy and Calibration of the Cardia    132

    5   The Guarner Partial Fundoplication    138

**VI** | *Strictures* **141**

    1   The Collis Gastroplasty and Antireflux Repair    142

    2   Thal Patch and Antireflux Repair    148

    3   Intrathoracic Total Fundoplication    150

**VII** | *Motor Disorders* **155**

    1   Achalasia    156

    2   Diffuse Esophageal Spasm    160

    3   Zenker's Diverticulum    162

    4   Epiphrenic Diverticulum    166

    5   Leiomyoma    172

**VIII** | *Esophageal Rupture* **175**

    1   Primary Repair with Pleural Patch    176

    2   Esophageal Diversion    180

*Index* **183**

# Operative Approaches to the Esophagus

The esophagus passes through three body regions, the neck, thorax, and upper abdomen, requiring the surgeon performing an esophageal operation to have knowledge and experience with the several incisions used to approach the esophagus. Frequently the incisions are used in combination in a single operation.

# 1 | *Abdominal Approaches*

**A**

Several abdominal incisions may be used to approach the abdominal esophagus and the hiatus. I prefer a right subcostal incision extended to the left costal margin in all patients except those whose costal cartilages and xiphoid form an acute angle where they meet. The extended right subcostal incision enables the use of the self-retaining broad "upper hand" retractor, and the multilayer closure has advantages for wound healing.

**B**

For those with a narrow costal margin, the midline incision from xiphoid to umbilicus may be used. An alternative which gives better exposure is to extend the midline incision to a point midway between the xiphoid and umbilicus and perform a transverse incision from one costal margin to the other at this level.

**C**

To perform the extended right subcostal approach, the skin incision is started lateral to the rectus sheath one fingerbreadth below the costal margin, crosses the midline just below the xiphoid process, and extends straight to the left costal margin. The external and internal oblique muscles and their fascia are incised to open the rectus sheath. The right rectus muscle is divided using cautery. The superior epigastric artery is ligated and divided. The incision is carried in a straight line across the linea alba, and the left rectus sheath is opened. The anterior and posterior aponeuroses enclosing the left rectus muscle are incised to the costal margin, but the muscle itself is simply retracted. Finally, the posterior rectus sheath or transversalis fascia is incised to expose the retroperitoneal fat and enter the peritoneum. The falciforme ligament is divided.

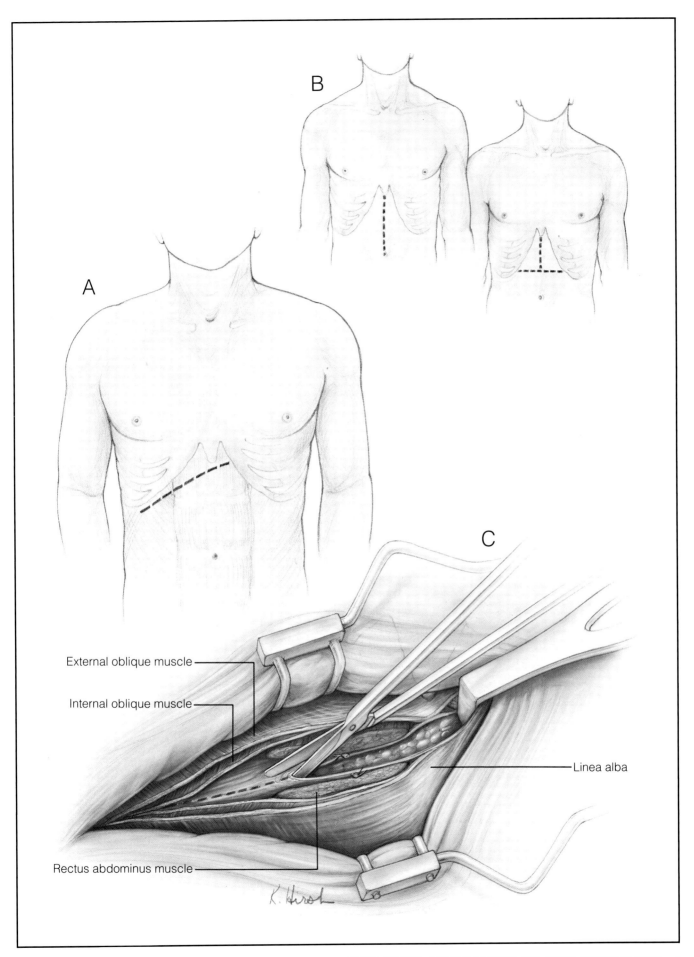

External oblique muscle

Internal oblique muscle

Rectus abdominus muscle

Linea alba

R. Hiroh

Exposure is first obtained using a Balfour self-retaining retractor. The left lobe of the liver is drawn down by placing the left index and middle fingers behind the triangular ligament. A small vessel in the margin is clamped. The ligament is divided to the right, stopping just short of the vena cava. Care is taken to avoid a phrenic vein coursing just cephalad and anterior to the triangular ligament and entering the inferior vena cava.

The Balfour retractor is removed, and a broad "upper hand" retractor is placed in the midline and attached to a sterile frame mounted to posts on the operating table. Strong upward retraction and fixation of this instrument provides excellent exposure of the hiatus. The left lobe of the liver is retracted to the right and protected by a gauze pad held by a Deaver retractor. Occasionally the left lobe of the liver is folded under to obtain this exposure, but this may create ischemic damage to the left lobe.

To expose the esophagus, the peritoneum and fascia on the anterior edge of the hiatus are incised from the reflection of the upper gastrohepatic ligament circumferentially around to the reflection of the peritoneum onto the gastric fundus. The hepatic branch of the vagus nerve is preserved in the upper portion of the gastrohepatic ligament.

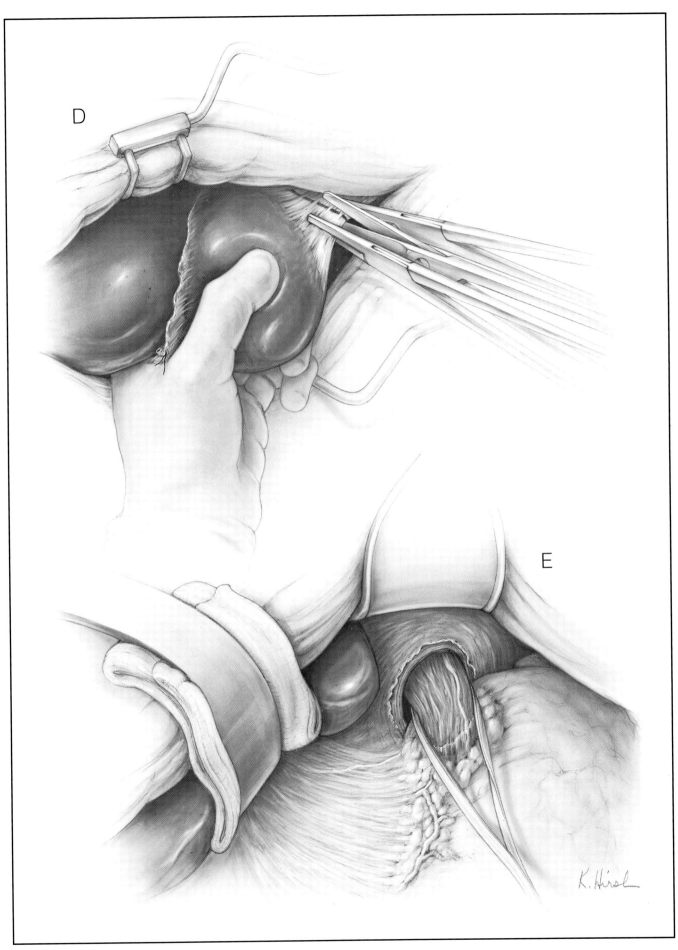

D

E

K. Hirsh

# 2 | *Thoracic Approach — Left Thoracotomy*

*A*

A left thoracotomy incision through the sixth interspace provides ideal exposure of the esophagus from the aortic arch to the hiatus. The patient's left arm is extended under tension by the anesthesiologist, and the skin incision is made from the posterior angle of the rib along the course of the seventh rib to the costal chondral junction anteriorly. The incision should not be curved upward nor should it extend onto the flat part of the back medial to the posterior angle of the rib to avoid wound problems resulting from the patient lying flat in bed on the incision. After the initial skin scalpel incision, electrocautery is used to deepen the thoracotomy.

*B*

The latissimus dorsi muscle is divided across its entire width making the incision as low as possible within the thoracotomy wound to preserve innervated muscle. The chest wall is approached posterior to the latissimus dorsi. A hand is passed under the scapula on the chest wall to the apex to obtain a more accurate counting of the ribs. If the surgeon does not push aggressively upward to the subclavicular region, it is assumed that the highest rib easily palpated is the second rib from which the surgeon begins to count to identify the sixth and seventh ribs. A cautery mark is placed on the superior aspect of the seventh rib. In operations for benign disease it is usually not necessary to divide the serratus anterior which is retracted anteriorly. The external intercostal muscle fibers are divided with cautery starting posteriorly at the margin of the paraspinal muscle mass and continuing the incision anteriorly. In this way, the direction of insertion of the intercostal muscles keeps the cautery tip applied to the superior margin of the seventh rib and minimizes bleeding. This intercostal incision can be carried underneath the serratus muscle to the costal chondral junction without difficulty. In more extensive operations, for malignant disease, it is frequently necessary to divide the serratus anterior muscle. A thoracoabdominal incision crossing the costal margin is no longer used for any of the standard esophageal operations for benign or malignant disease.

*C*

Once the intercostal muscles are separated from the seventh rib, a segment of the rib is exposed beneath the paraspinal muscles. Using cautery, the erector spinous muscle is lifted off the seventh rib and elevated from the top of the eighth rib up to the sixth rib. A retractor is placed under the paraspinal muscle mass to expose the neck of the rib posterior to the angle. The periosteum is cleared for a 2-cm distance in this region using a periostal elevator and a Doyen rib periosteal elevator to avoid damage to the seventh intercostal bundle. Once the rib is completely isolated a 1-cm segment is resected beneath the paraspinal muscles to allow the rib to be folded inferiorly without causing a rib fracture. This diminishes postoperative pain. Unless injured by the dissection, the intercostal bundle is left intact. The pleura is entered.

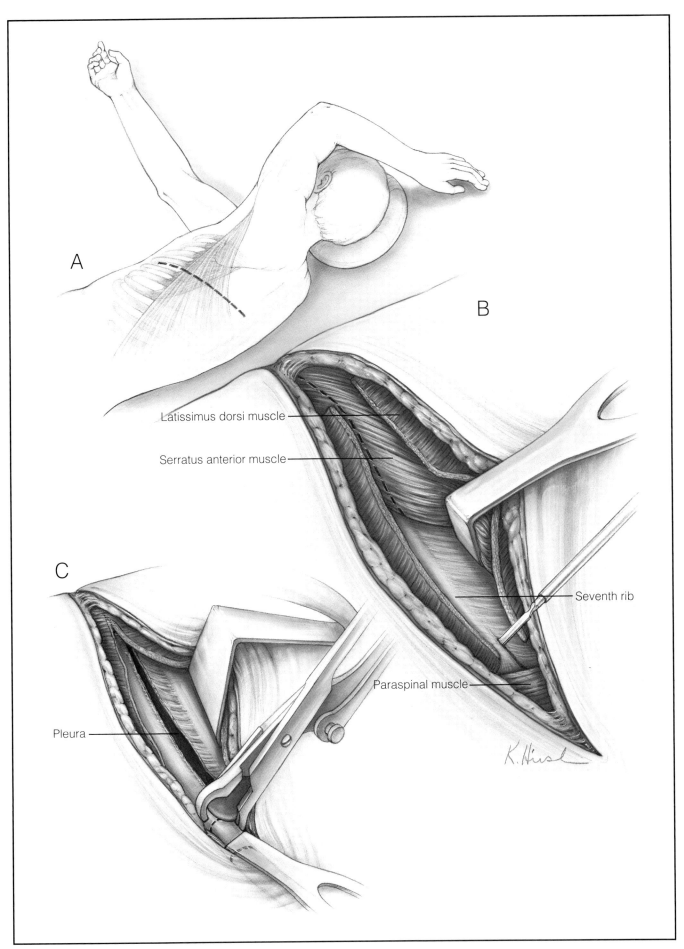

A

B

Latissimus dorsi muscle

Serratus anterior muscle

Seventh rib

Paraspinal muscle

C

Pleura

K. Hirsh

The thoracotomy is opened gradually with gentle pressure applied to the sixth and seventh ribs. I prefer to use a Balfour retractor with shallow blades to open the thoracotomy instead of the Finochietto rib spreader. By opening the Balfour with finger pressure, excess force which may lead to rib fractures is avoided. The thoracotomy should be opened only enough to permit access to the posterior mediastinum.

The first maneuver in approaching the esophagus is to divide the pulmonary ligament. There is frequently a small vessel near the free margin which is clamped and ligated to avoid intraoperative or postoperative bleeding. The ligament is incised from its free margin up to the inferior pulmonary vein. Frequently, another small vessel is found just beneath the pulmonary vein which again requires clamping and ligation.

The lung is retracted anteriorly and superiorly to expose the posterior mediastinum. The incised pleura along the base of the pulmonary ligament is dissected anteriorly and posteriorly to expose the muscle of the esophagus when it is being mobilized for benign disease. Using blunt dissection, the esophagus is gently elevated from its bed taking care to dissect the downside right pleura away from the longitudinal muscle which arises or inserts into subpleural fibrous tissue at this level. If the right pleura can be left intact, it avoids the accumulation of blood in the right pleural cavity that may lead to underestimation of operative blood loss and the need for postoperative right as well as left chest tubes. The esophagus is lifted from its bed dissecting away the right pleura down to the level of the hiatus. At least one and sometimes several esophageal or esophagobronchial arteries must be divided passing from the medial aspect of the aorta to the esophagus.

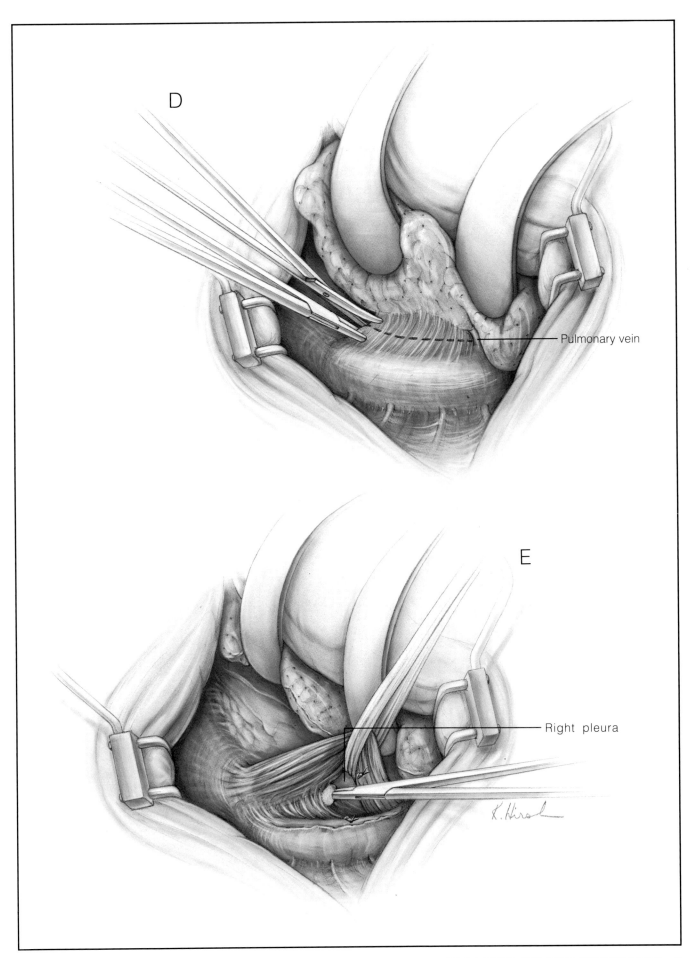

D

Pulmonary vein

E

Right pleura

K. Hirok

# 3 | *Thoracic Approach— Right Thoracotomy*

**A** A right thoracotomy is preferred for lesions of the middle third of the esophagus to avoid the interference of the aortic arch with the exposure. The incision is made over the right fifth interspace between the fifth and sixth ribs. Again, strong upward pull on the right arm is essential to move the scapula out of the region of the thoracotomy. The layers are divided in a manner similar to that described for the left thoracotomy. A posterior 1-cm segment of sixth rib is resected.

**B** Once the pleura is opened and the Balfour retractor inserted, the pulmonary ligament is divided up to the level of the pulmonary vein, and the lung is retracted anterior and superiorly. The esophagus is readily seen attached to the right pleura. The pleura is incised to the extent necessary for the proposed procedure. In this illustration, an esophageal tumor is being exposed, and the esophagus is elevated off the aorta taking care to avoid entry into the left pleural cavity. When necessary, the azygos arch can be divided.

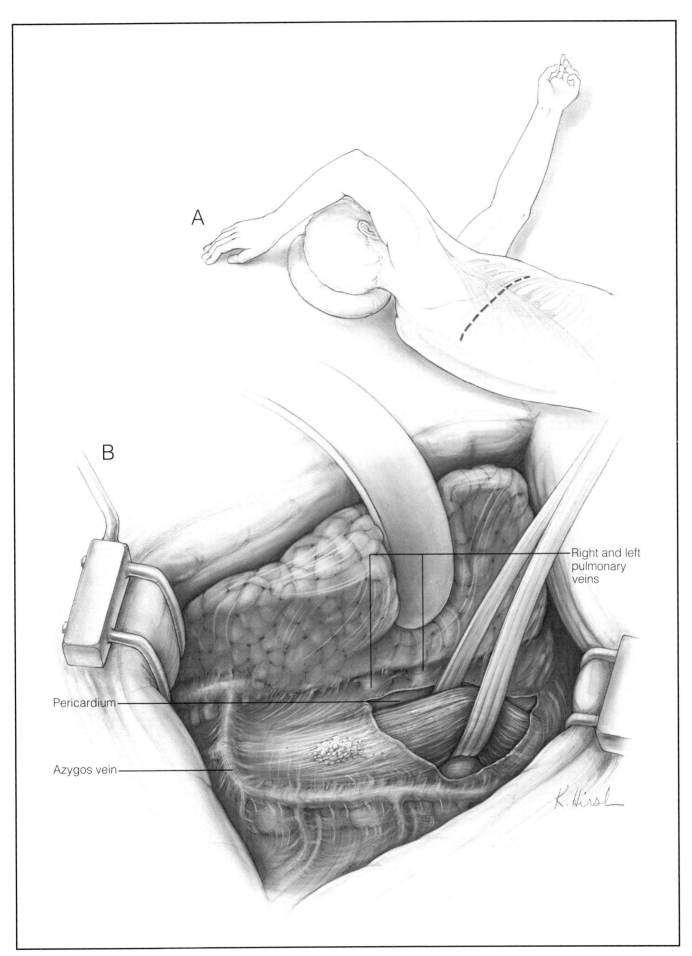

A

B

Right and left pulmonary veins

Pericardium

Azygos vein

K. Hirsl

# 4 | Approaches to the Cervical Esophagus

The cervical esophagus can be approached through either the right or left side of the neck depending on the purpose of the operation.

 A transverse collar incision is made approximately 1 fingerbreadth above the clavicle. In this case a right cervical approach is illustrated. The incision extends from the medial edge of the left sternocleidomastoid muscle across the midline to the lateral border of the right sterno-cleidomastoid muscle. After the incision is deepened through the platysma, skin flaps are elevated between the platysma and the fascia overlying the sternocleidomastoid and strap muscles. The superior flap is elevated to the level of the cricoid cartilage and the inferior flap to the level of the sternal notch and clavicles.

 The skin flaps are elevated with a self-retaining retractor. An incision is made in the groove where the fascia comes off the sternocleidomastoid muscle onto the sternohyoid muscle.

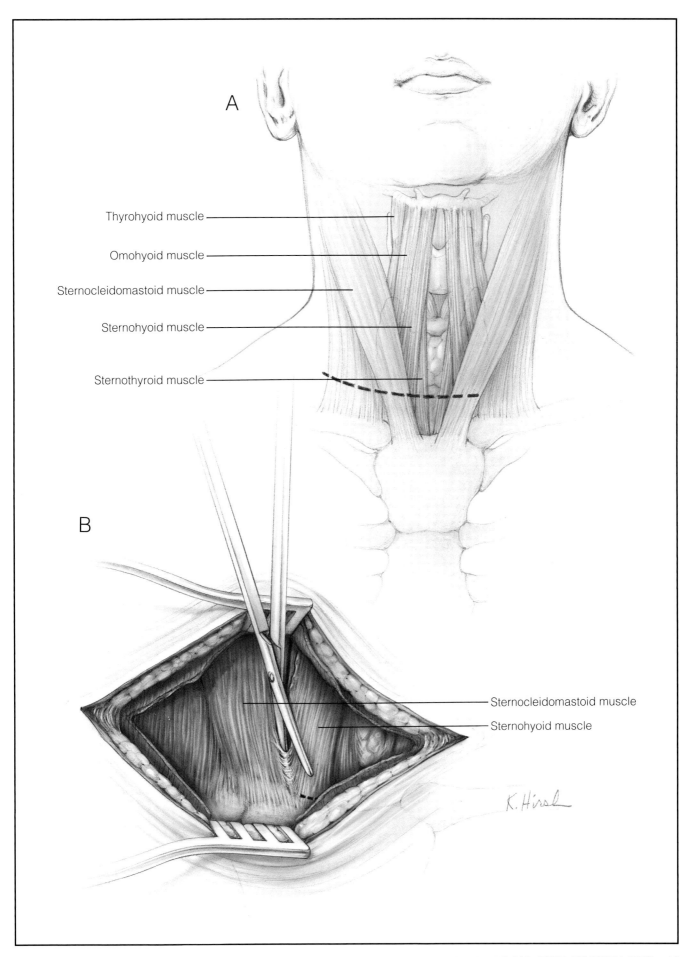

Thyrohyoid muscle

Omohyoid muscle

Sternocleidomastoid muscle

Sternohyoid muscle

Sternothyroid muscle

A

B

Sternocleidomastoid muscle

Sternohyoid muscle

K. Hirsh

C Once the plane between the strap muscles and sternocleidomastoid is developed, it is deepened medial to the carotid and jugular vessels to the prevertebral fascia. A mid-thyroid vein frequently crosses this dissection and is ligated and divided. When the prevertebral space is entered, it is readily dissected up and down between the posterior esophagus and the vertebral bodies.

At no time is a retractor applied to the medial portion of the deep incision. This avoids injury to the recurrent laryngeal nerve in the tracheoesophageal groove. To provide the necessary retraction medially, a deep figure of eight suture is placed through the strap muscles and into the underlying thyroid gland and pulled medially to provide rotation and retraction that will expose the right lateral wall of the esophagus.

C

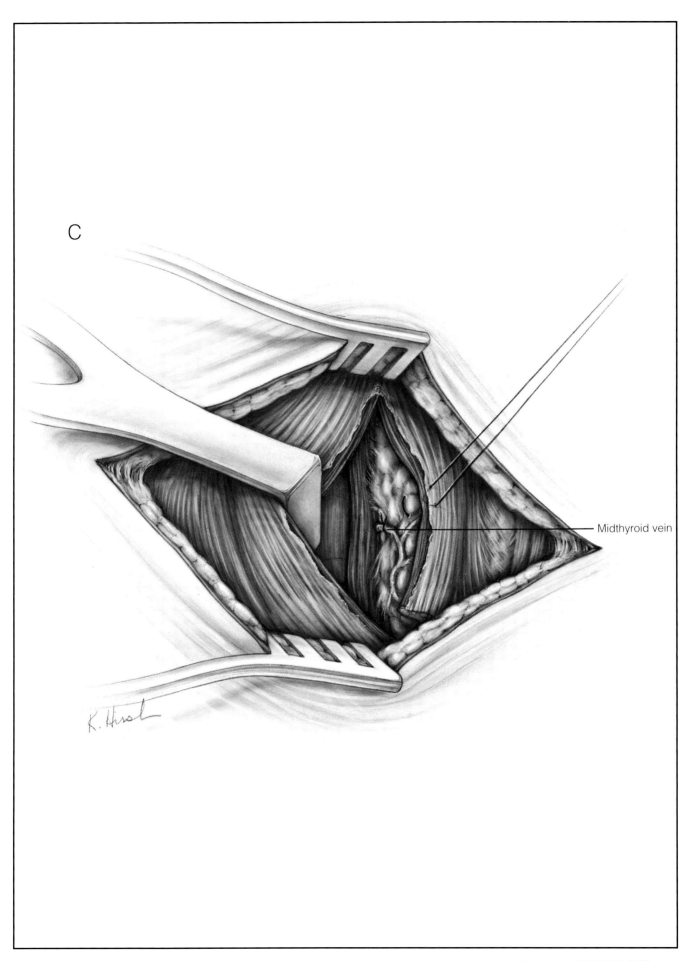

Midthyroid vein

K. Hirsch

# 5 | Cervical Approach Combined With Partial Sternotomy

*A*

For neoplasms of the cervical esophagus or thoracic inlet, better exposure for a thorough dissection is obtained by adding a partial median sternotomy to the previously described cervical incision. A partial instead of total sternotomy is preferred to maintain stability of the sternum. Because operations on the esophagus introduce the risk of contamination with mouth or intestinal flora, the chance for an infected total sternotomy incision is greater than for cardiac surgery. This risk is minimized if the sternum is left with its distal portion intact.

The sternal incision is carried across the manubrium and down to approximately the insertion of the third costal cartilage. After the cervical incision is opened, a midline extension of the skin incision is made to this point. The substernal space is cleared bluntly and a vibrating saw with a bullet nose to protect deep tissue divides the sternum. Alternatively an oscillating saw may be used. The incision is kept to the midline to facilitate placement of closure sutures.

*B*

A Tuffier retractor is used with one aspect of the sternal incision retracted anteriorly and the other somewhat posteriorly as in a clam shell opening. This provides exposure to the underlying confluence of the left and right jugular veins into the innominate vein and the innominate artery coming off the aortic arch. These may be retracted laterally to provide excellent exposure of the esophagus in the thoracic inlet and enable the performance of a lymph node dissection should this be desired. It may be necessary to remove the thymus gland and ligate its vein entering the innominate vein. The strap muscles are divided from the posterior aspects of the sternum which is critical to opening the thoracic inlet.

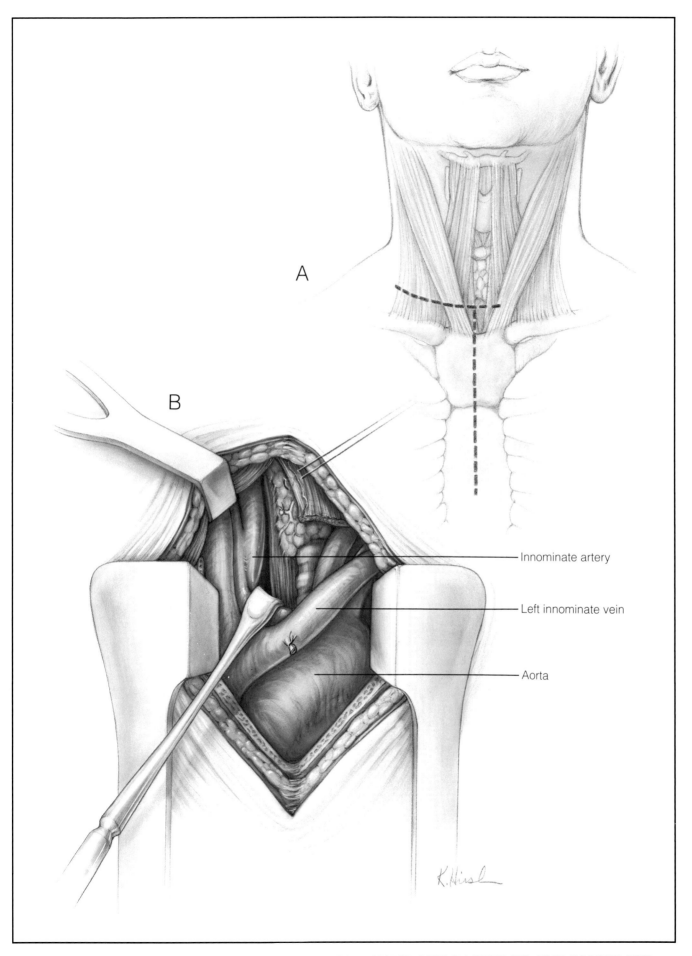

A

B

Innominate artery

Left innominate vein

Aorta

K. Hirsh

# CHAPTER II

# Resection for Malignant Neoplasms

Several approaches may be used for resection of esophageal carcinoma depending on the location of the tumor and whether the intent of the operation is curative as determined through staging, or palliative to relieve dysphagia and tumor complications. When preoperative staging including CT scan analysis, endoscopy preferably with ultrasound, and overall evaluation of the patient suggests the neoplasm is limited to the esophageal wall and without enlarged distal lymph nodes, an en bloc resection of the esophagus in the region of the tumor is performed to obtain an envelope of tissue surrounding the esophagus for maximal local control. When preoperative staging suggests that cure is unlikely because of penetration beyond the esophagus or enlarged lymph nodes, a standard or palliative esophagectomy dissecting adjacent to the wall of the esophagus and removing obviously enlarged lymph nodes is performed to relieve dysphagia and tumor complications. Esophagectomy without thoracotomy may be used for palliation except for bulky tumors in the region of the carina and aortic arch where the procedure may be unsafe. Esophagectomy without thoracotomy is used in conjunction with curative resections for tumors of the cervical esophagus or intra-abdominal esophagus in which removal of the intrathoracic esophagus is desired before reconstruction.

# 1 | *En Bloc Esophagectomy Through a Left Thoracotomy*

**A**  A schematic cross-section of the thorax at the level of the seventh thoracic vertebra is shown. In the embryo, the esophagus distal to the aortic arch is suspended from a mesoesophagus, as is the rest of the digestive tract. Accordingly, the lymphatic and vascular structures approach the esophagus dorsally. In the adult, the venous drainage goes to the azygos vein and the lymphatic drainage to the thoracic duct. Longitudinal muscle fibers in the thoracic esophagus arise or insert from subpleural and subpericardial fibrous tissue that lies adjacent to the esophagus. In effect, the pericardial and pleural surfaces act as a serosa to the esophagus. The concept of total removal of the thoracic esophagus for attempted cure includes resection of the overlying pericardium and pleura as well as the dorsal tissues between the esophagus and vertebral bodies as the esophageal mesentery. By performing this resection en bloc, the actual muscular wall of the esophagus is not seen during the resection until the wall is approached at the point for transection.

**B**  After completion of the en bloc resection, the remaining structures adjacent to the posterior mediastinum are the anterior vertebral bodies, aorta, myocardium, and right and left lungs.

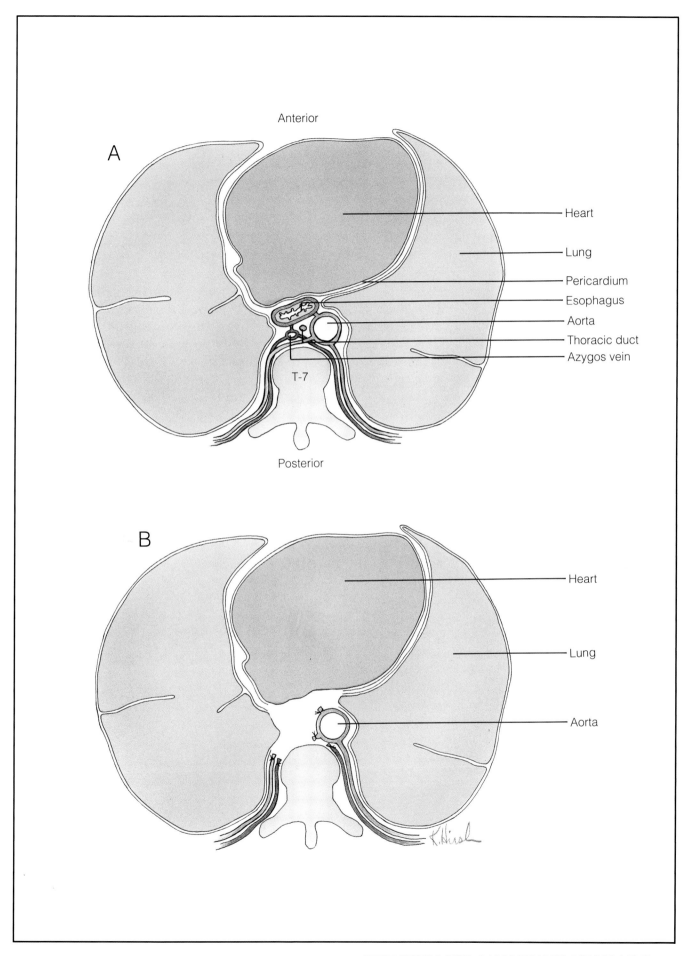

**C** For neoplasms arising 10 cm or more distal to the aortic arch pulsation measured endoscopically, the en bloc esophagectomy is performed through a left sixth interspace thoracotomy as previously illustrated. For this resection the serratus muscle is divided so that the intercostal space is widely opened between the sixth and seventh costal cartilages. The costal margin is not divided. It is not necessary to remove a rib since the posterior seventh rib transection allows this rib to be folded back by the Balfour chest wall retractor.

**D** After the pulmonary ligament is divided and the vessel (Sweet's artery) at the base of the inferior pulmonary vein is ligated and divided, the pericardial sheath over the pulmonary veins is exposed. Dotted lines denote the eventual extent of the pleural, pericardial, and diaphragmatic incisions. The diaphragm will be detached from the chest wall peripherally under the rib cage as indicated by the dotted line.

**E** The pleura under the aortic arch and on the back of the left main stem bronchus is incised so that a lymph node in this region may be biopsied. Since these nodes are approximately 10 cm from the tumor, a positive lymph node on frozen section at this location indicates that the patient is unlikely to be cured by the en bloc resection. If this proves to be the case, a palliative resection performed on the wall of the esophagus is undertaken instead of the originally planned more extensive en bloc resection.

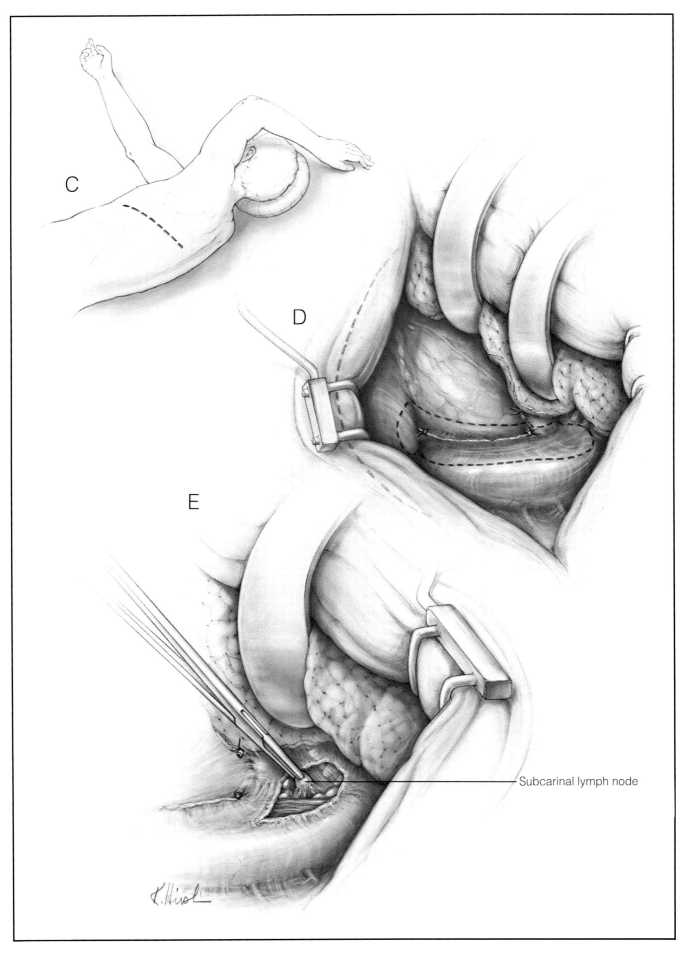

C

D

E

Subcarinal lymph node

Viewing the diaphragm from below, the location for the incision of the diaphragm made through a left thoracotomy is indicated by the dotted line. The incision starts medially under the sternum and is carried circumferentially to the posterior margin of the palpable spleen. Approximately a 1 inch cuff of diaphragm muscle is left attached to the chest wall for subsequent reattachments.

With the diaphragm open and retracted, the spleen, splenic flexure, and entire left upper quadrant are readily exposed. The omentum is elevated out of the abdomen through the thoracotomy incision. Embryologically, the omentum fuses with the mesocolon resulting in an avascular plane between these two structures. This plane can be entered by separating the omentum from its adherence to the splenic flexure and transverse colon and then peeling the omental tissues away from the mesocolon. Usually no vessels are encountered until the region of the hepatic flexure is reached. Colonic vessels in the mesocolon tend to be tented up as the omentum is pulled away, and care must be taken to leave these vessels behind in the mesocolon and on the colonic wall. As the omentum is elevated off the mesocolon, the lesser sac is penetrated near the base of the omentum.

Once the entire omentum is mobilized over to the hepatic flexure and the lesser sac opened, the stomach is reflected superiorly. This exposes the pancreas in the region of the celiac axis. A lymph node at this location, which represents the furthest extent of the resection, is biopsied and sent for frozen section. A positive node at this location suggests incurability, and a decision is made to do a palliative resection. Assuming the node biopsy is negative, the dissection is carried from the celiac access along the splenic artery. If the spleen is closely adjacent to the tumor as in the case illustrated, a splenectomy is carried out. Otherwise the left gastroepiploic vessels and short gastric vessels between the splenic artery and stomach are divided, but the spleen is left intact.

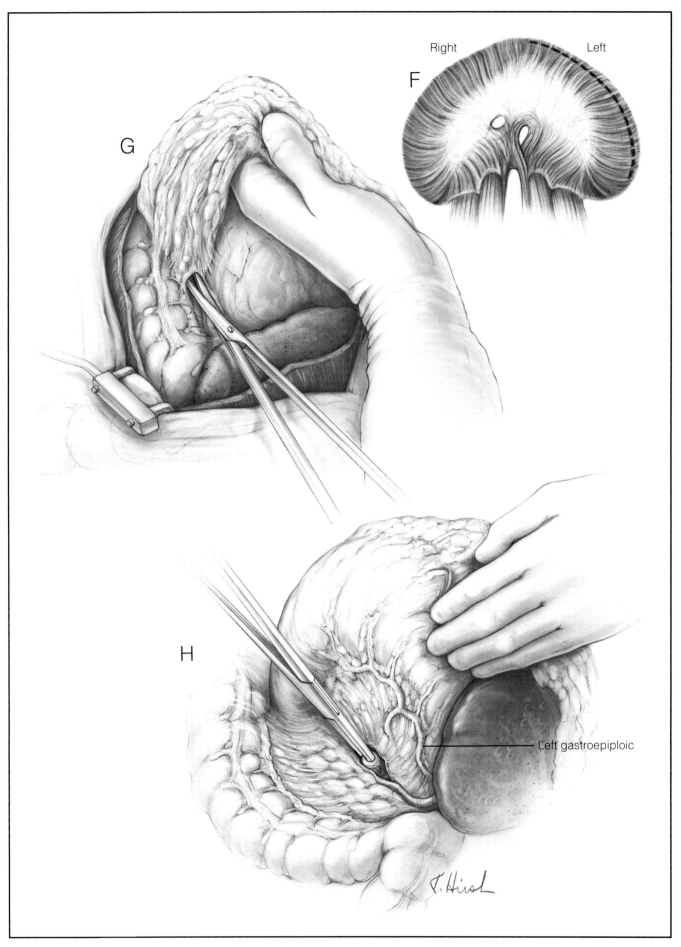

F
Right                    Left

G

H

Left gastroepiploic

T. Hirsh

*I*  Dissection of the branches of the celiac artery is complete. The coronary vein is ligated and divided anteriorly and to the right of the left gastric artery. The left gastric artery is exposed, ligated, and divided at its origin from the celiac artery. The tissues surrounding the left gastric trunk are dissected upward with the specimen to be removed. The dissection is carried onto the origins of the diaphragm off the arcuate ligament, and all of the retroperitoneal tissues cephalad to the celiac axis are swept up toward the hiatus and included in the resection.

*J*  After the retroperitoneal tissues are brought into the region of the hiatus, the muscles surrounding the hiatus are divided by electrocautery to provide a cuff of diaphragm surrounding the tumor in the region of the hiatus. A left inferior phrenic artery arising from the left adrenal artery crosses close to the hiatus and requires ligation and division. Once the diaphragm muscles around the hiatus are detached circumferentially, the posterior mediastinum is entered. The aorta is retracted to the left exposing the origins of the thoracic duct where lymphatics from the cisterna chyla converge. The duct is doubly ligated at this level and divided. The origin of the azygos vein is found on the vertebral body where the ascending lumbar veins converge. This is similarly ligated and divided. The abdominal portion of the en bloc mobilization is complete.

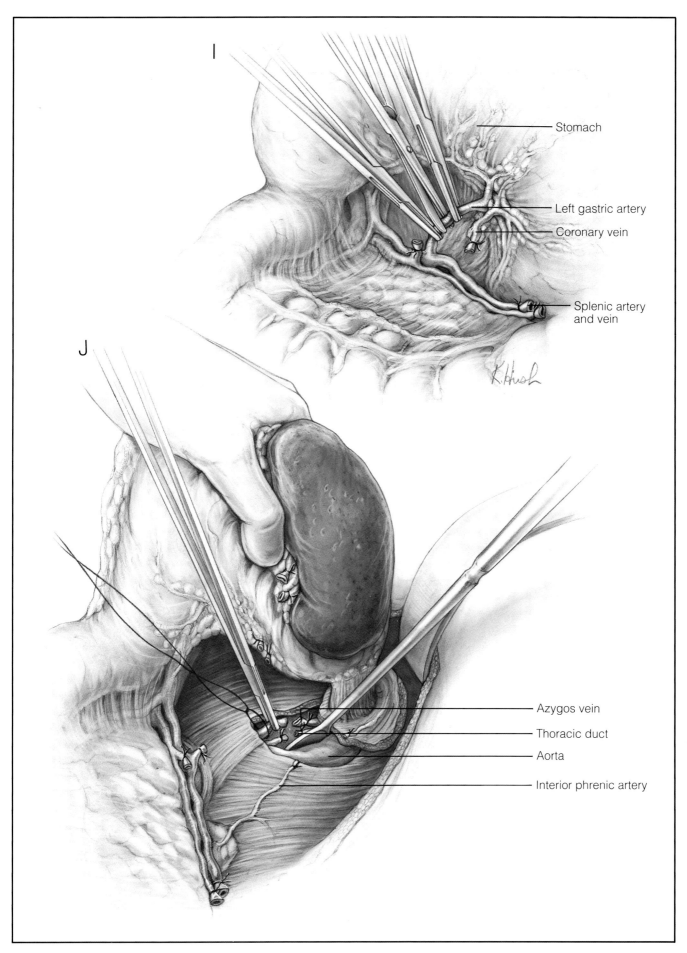

I

Stomach

Left gastric artery

Coronary vein

Splenic artery
and vein

J

Azygos vein

Thoracic duct

Aorta

Interior phrenic artery

The diaphragm is retracted inferiorly to expose the mediastinum again. The diaphragm incised around the hiatus opens the lower posterior mediastinum. An incision is made along the descending aorta until the aortic arch is reached. One or more esophageal or esophago-bronchial arteries are ligated and divided on the aorta. Periaortic tissues are swept medially toward the esophagus. This region is the site of many lymphatics, and the larger ones should be ligated to reduce postoperative chest tube drainage.

On the vertebral column medial to the aorta, the left intercostal veins and right intercostal arteries are ligated and divided to expose the vertebral body. By elevating these tissues the mesoesophagus including the azygos vein and thoracic duct are brought up with the esophagus. The dissection is carried to the right side of the vertebral body where the right intercostal arteries and veins are again ligated and divided as they pass posteriorly to the right intercostal spaces. This dissection is carried proximally until the desired 10-cm margin above the palpable tumor is reached, usually just distal to the aortic arch.

After division of the intercostal vessels and clearing of the vertebral body, the right pleural cavity is entered posterior to the right pulmonary ligament to leave the right pleura adherent to the esophagus in the region of the tumor. On the back of the superior pulmonary vein, the pericardium is entered. A pericardial incision is made from this point to the diaphragm along the reflection of the left pleura off the pericardium. By applying traction on the pericardium adherent to the esophagus in the region of the pulmonary veins, the exit of the right pulmonary veins from the pericardium is identified, and an incision is made at this point from inside the pericardium into the right pleural cavity. This incision will come out in front of the right pulmonary ligament. The incision in the pericardium on the right side is carried down to the diaphragm where it joins the left pericardial incision. Now the only remaining attachment of the esophagus enclosed within its envelope of surrounding tissues is the right pulmonary ligament, which is divided under direct vision by elevating the specimen up into the left thorax.

K

L

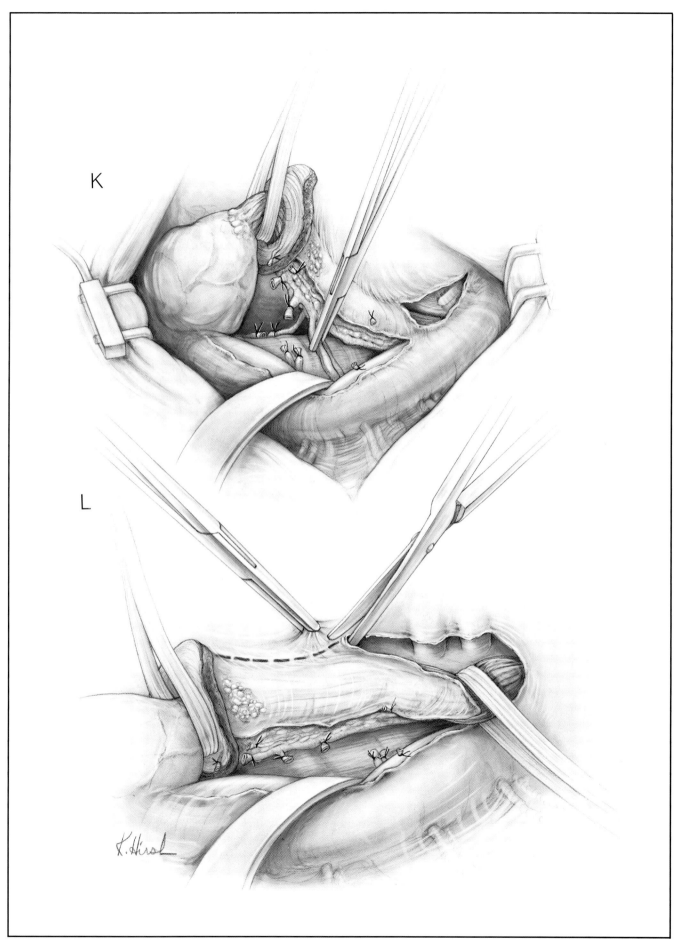

K. Hirsh

The en bloc mobilization of the esophagus is now complete. The aorta and the stumps of the intercostal vessels passing into the right chest are carefully inspected for hemostasis. The defect in the pericardium is sufficiently large to avoid problems with a heart hernia, and allows the pericardium to remain widely open. The right lung is visible in the depths of the field. At the end of the procedure a right chest tube is inserted before the patient is removed from the operating room.

With this surgical procedure the tumor in the distal esophagus is completely enclosed within pleura, pericardium, and mesoesophagus, and the actual muscular wall of the esophagus is only seen at the level of the aortic arch where the desired 10-cm margin is achieved. The stage is now set for removal of this specimen including 10 cm of the lesser curvature of the stomach below the tumor and a similar amount on the greater curvature. If the neoplasm is an adenocarcinoma, and squamous epithelium is present at the resection margin, reconstruction can be made just below the aortic arch. If the tumor is a squamous cell carcinoma or there is Barrett's esophagus at the resection margin, the dissection is carried under the aortic arch and a reconstruction made in the neck. The steps for reconstruction are described in Chapter III.

M

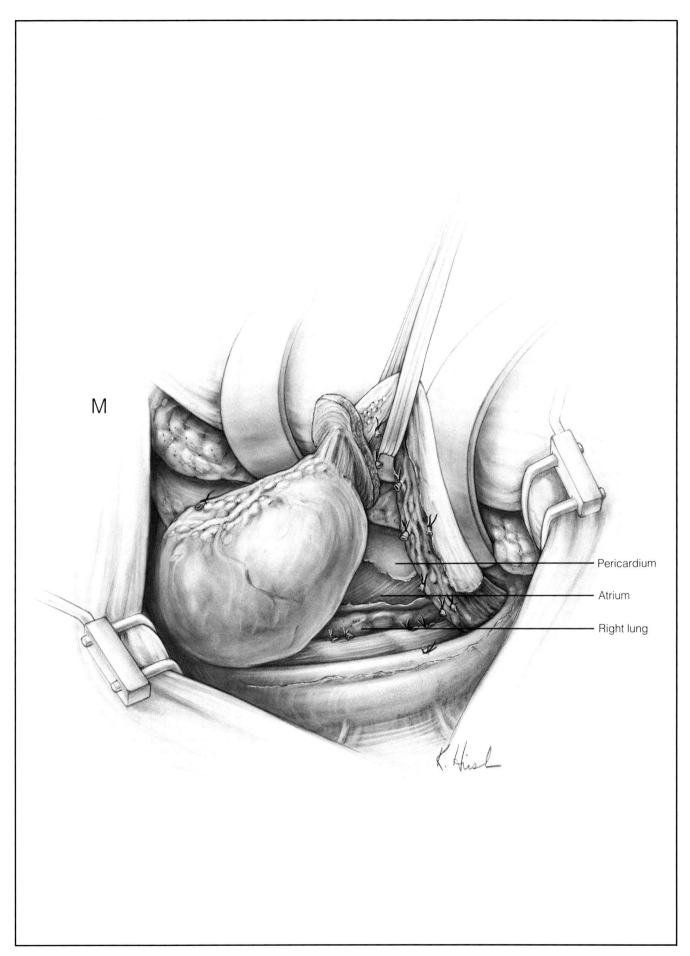

Pericardium

Atrium

Right lung

# 2 | *En Bloc Esophagectomy Through a Right Thoracotomy*

**A**

For tumors that are located closer than 10 cm to the aortic arch, a right thoracotomy is performed for en bloc resection of the intrathoracic esophagus. The incision is made in the fifth interspace and enters the pleura on top of the sixth rib.

**B**

The right intercostal arteries and veins are ligated and divided as they pass from the vertebral body to the right chest wall. This opens the plane on the anterior surface of the vertebral body and begins the elevation of the azygos vein and thoracic duct. Anteriorly the azygos vein is divided and oversewn flush with the vena cava. The pleura is incised on the lateral aspect of the trachea, over the right main bronchus onto the back of the right pulmonary veins. The pericardium is incised from the superior vein down to the level of the diaphragm. The left pericardial incision is made by retracting the pericardium to the right in order to see the exit of the left pulmonary veins from the pericardium. The pericardial patch is resected in a manner similar to that described for the left thoracic approach. The dissection is carried across the vertebral body to the aorta where the right intercostal arteries and left intercostal veins are ligated and divided. The left pleura is opened just in front of the aorta. Lastly, the left pulmonary ligament is incised under direct vision.

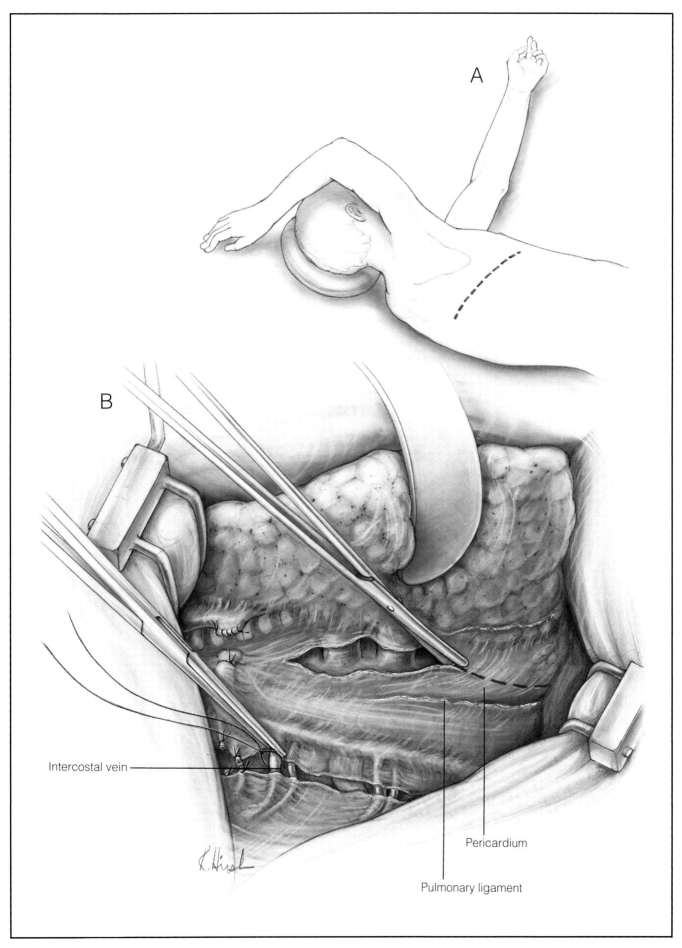

A

B

Intercostal vein

Pericardium

Pulmonary ligament

The completed en bloc resection through a right thoracotomy is shown with pleural, and pericardial tissue overlying the esophagus and a resection of the posterior mesoesophagus. Reconstruction can be performed by advancing the stomach through the hiatus as described on pages 40 and 41 or by preparation of the stomach or colon through a separate laparotomy incision. With this approach, the anastomosis for the reconstruction is almost always made through a right cervical incision.

 A transverse section of the extent of the en bloc resection illustrated in the specimen above is shown with the points of transection of the various structures indicated.

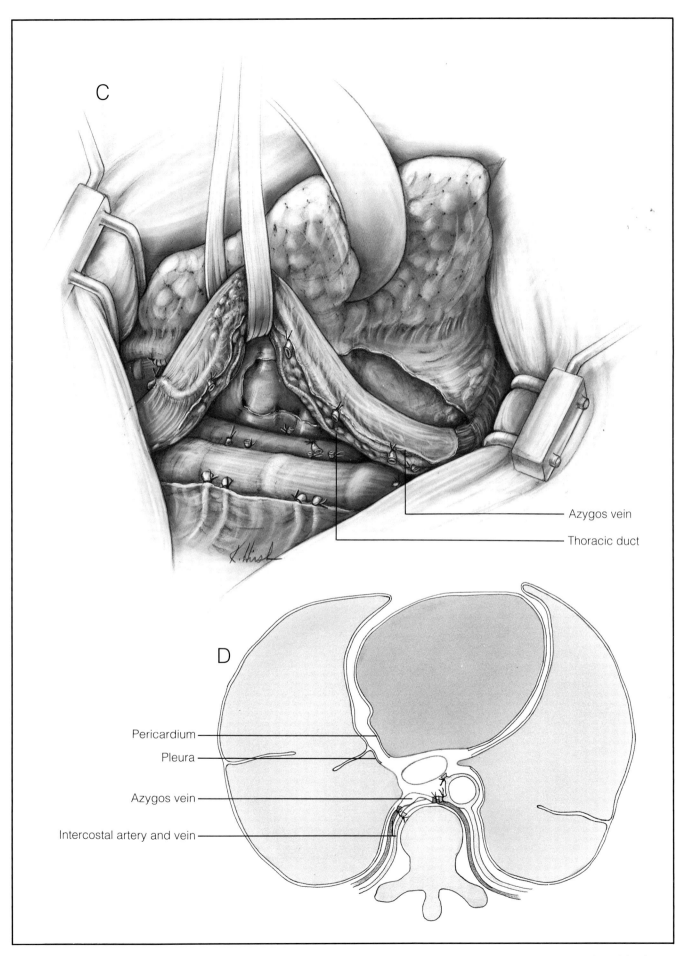

C

Azygos vein

Thoracic duct

D

Pericardium

Pleura

Azygos vein

Intercostal artery and vein

# 3 | Standard or Palliative Esophagectomy Through a Right Thoracotomy

*A*

For tumors of the midportion of the esophagus, a standard resection is performed through a right fifth interspace thoracotomy entering the pleura on the superior margin of the sixth rib.

*B*

After division of the pulmonary ligament, the esophagus is mobilized leaving as much tissue adjacent to the tumor as possible without entering the pericardium or resecting the mesoesophagus including the thoracic duct and azygos vein. In this illustration, the tumor is penetrating the pleura at the level of the right inferior pulmonary vein. A patch of pleural tissue is left on the specimen by incising the pleura in the pleuro-pericardial groove. The azygos arch is divided flush with the superior vena cava and is interrupted at the point of insertion of the highest intercostal vein. The esophagus is mobilized off the aorta with aortic vessels divided, but the intercostal vessels are not divided in a standard esophagectomy.

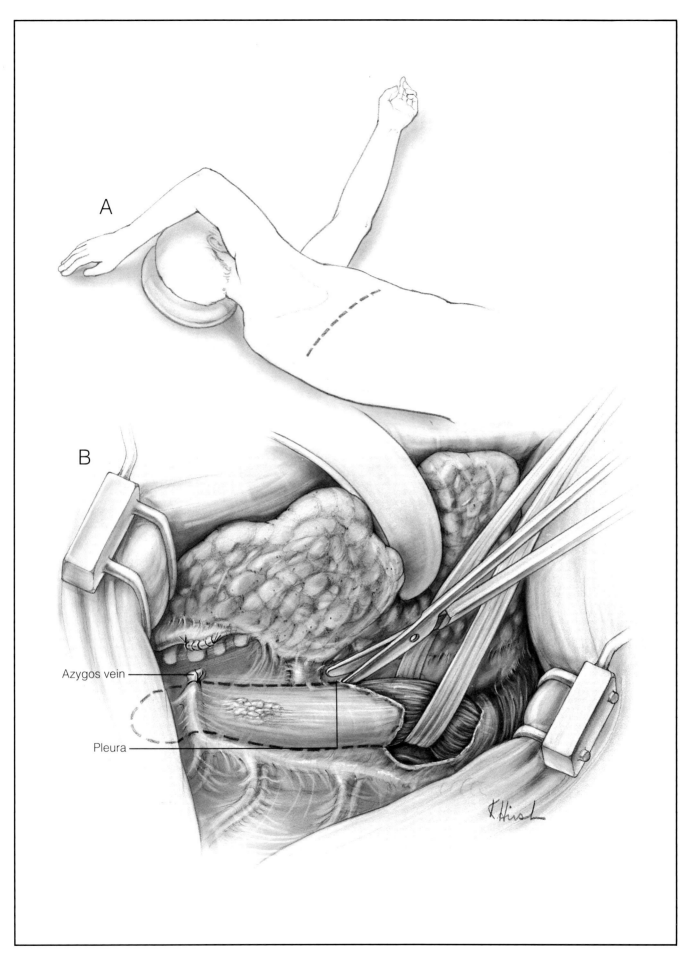

A

B

Azygos vein

Pleura

The esophagus is mobilized off the aorta, pericardium, and posterior tissues. The phrenoesophageal membrane is incised and drawn up into the thorax by tension on the esophagus.

 The incision passes through pleura overlying the muscular cuff of the hiatus, the endothoracic and endoabdominal fascia which create the phrenoesophageal membrane, and finally peritoneum to enter the abdomen.

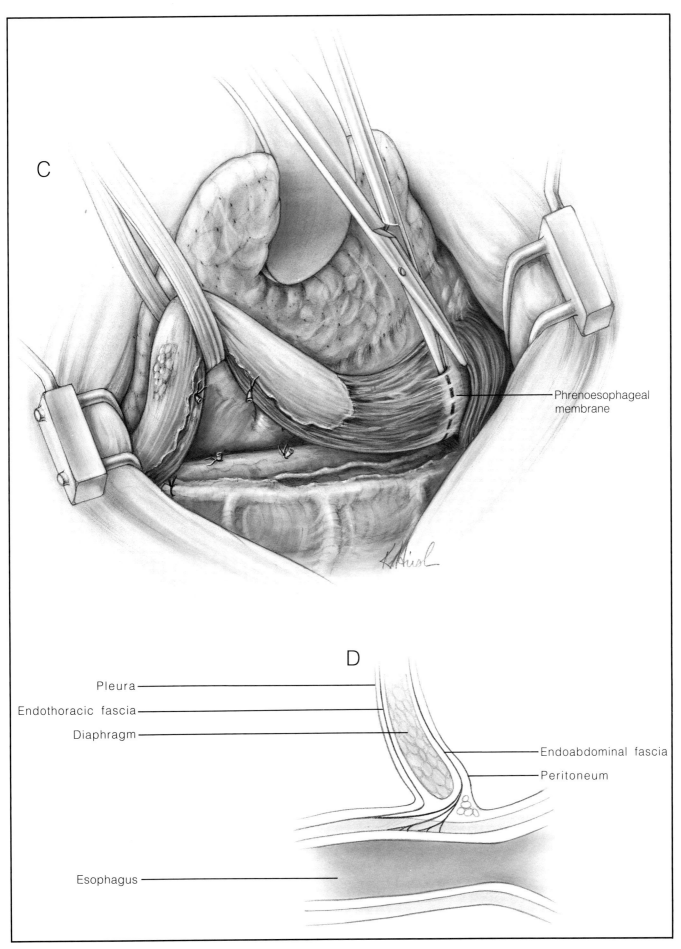

C

Phrenoesophageal
membrane

D

Pleura

Endothoracic fascia

Diaphragm

Endoabdominal fascia

Peritoneum

Esophagus

In patients who have not had prior abdominal surgery and who are not unduly obese, it is possible to mobilize the stomach through the hiatus without performing a separate laparotomy for reconstruction. This is especially attractive for patients receiving a palliative resection in which there is no concern about sampling intra-abdominal lymph nodes, and in those patients in whom preoperative or operative conditions dictate shortening the operation. The diagram shows the vessels to be divided through the hiatus. With finger dissection under the diaphragm, the highest short gastric vessels and the ascending branch of the left gastric artery are drawn up into the hiatus to begin the resection.

 With the esophagus drawn up under tension, the vessels present one after another into the hiatus. The vessels are doubly clamped on the distal side and doubly ligated to be certain that there is no intra-abdominal bleeding.

After the last of the left gastroepiploic vessels as well as the left gastric vessels are divided, the stomach comes up rather easily. The omentum is separated outside of the right gastroepiploic arcade to preserve blood supply to the stomach. In this fashion, the entire stomach down to the level of the pylorus can be delivered through the hiatus. In palliative cases, the anastomosis is made at least 5, preferably 10 cm proximal to the tumor in the apex of the chest. If the margin appears inadequate, the fundus of the stomach is temporarily attached to the closed esophagus at the apex of the chest, and the anastomosis is done through a separate cervical incision. In this type of resection for a midthoracic tumor, only the cardia is resected so that the whole stomach is used for the reconstruction.

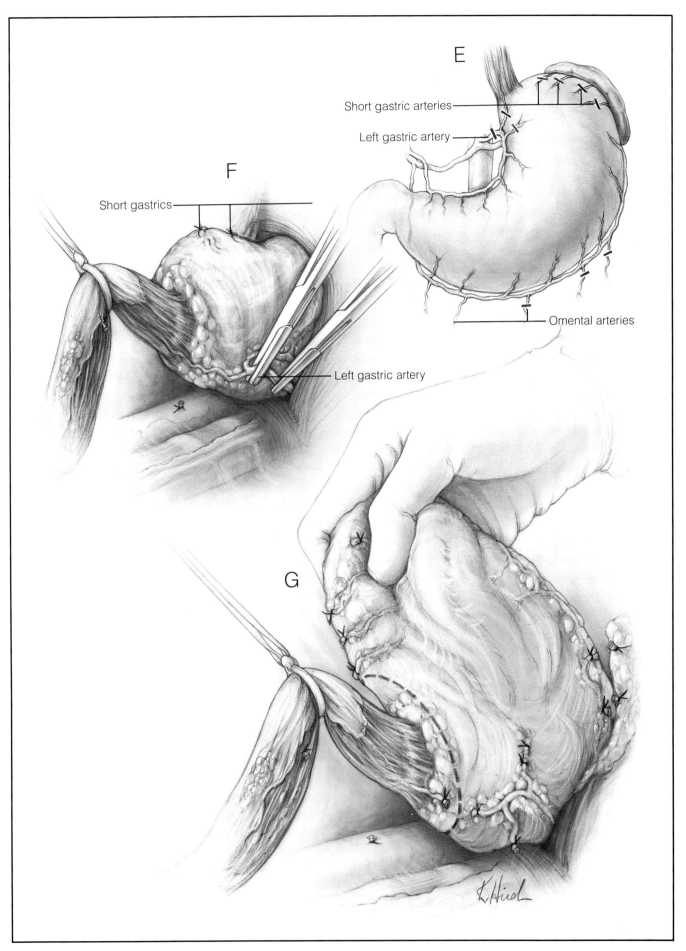

E

Short gastric arteries

Left gastric artery

Omental arteries

F

Short gastrics

Left gastric artery

G

# 4 | *Esophagectomy Without Thoracotomy*

In this patient resection is being performed for an adenocarcinoma of the distal intra-abdominal segment of esophagus. Steps similar to those taken in the transthoracic en bloc resection can be employed.

The right subcostal incision extended across the xiphoid to the left costal margin with use of the "upper hand" retractor provides excellent exposure. A right cervical incision is made.

**B** The resection is started by excising a cuff of diaphragm surrounding the hiatus with electrocautery to give some additional local margin around the tumor and to provide access to the mediastinum. The high gastrohepatic ligament is divided close to the liver. In this illustration a left hepatic artery branch is seen coming from the esophageal branch of the left gastric artery. This is a fairly common anomaly. Unless this is an unusually large vessel, it can be divided without concern for liver function.

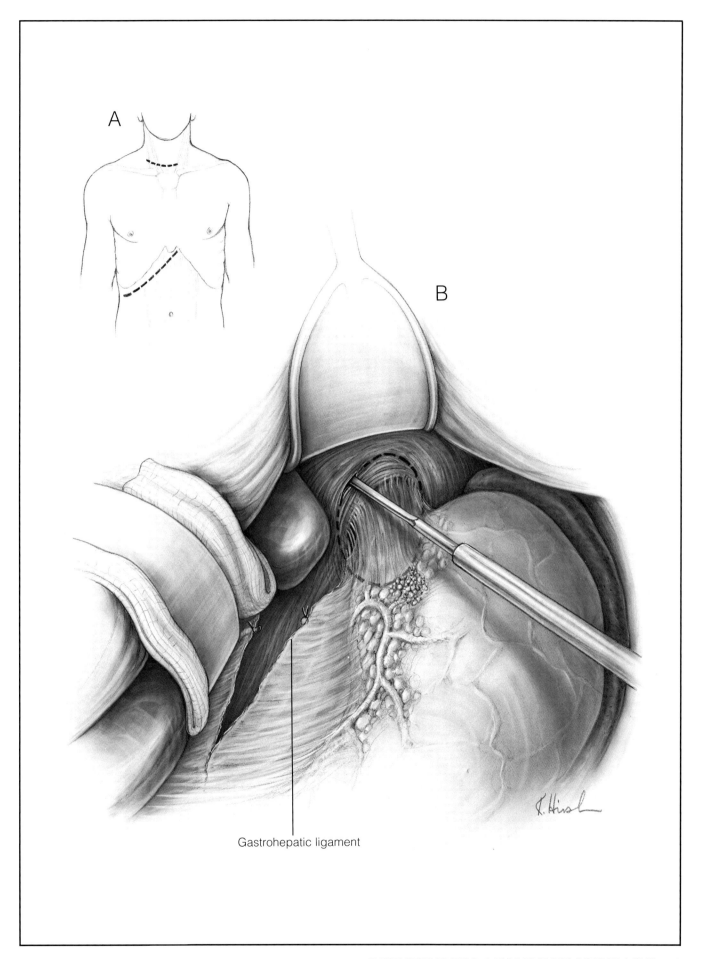

A

B

Gastrohepatic ligament

**C** With the stomach retracted to the left, the lesser sac is well seen. The coronary vein is ligated, and the origin of the left gastric artery is exposed and clamped at the celiac axis. As with the en bloc resection through a left thoracotomy, the tissues between the celiac axis and the cut margins of the hiatus are swept up with the esophagus and stomach specimen. Through the opened hiatus, the right pleura is seen and can be readily incised to leave a pleural attachment adjacent to the esophagus. Similarly, the azygos vein and thoracic duct can be ligated and divided at their origins if the tumor extends into the muscular tunnel of the hiatus.

**D** The left pleura can also be incised as it reflects off the diaphragm and remains attached to the esophagus. This provides excellent exposure of the anterior surface of the aorta. One or more esophageal arteries can be ligated and divided under direct vision through the hiatus. In this fashion the dissection may be carried up to 10 cm above the tumor staying on the surface of the aorta and vertebral bodies. At the highest point where exposure is still satisfactory, the azygos vein and thoracic duct are again ligated and divided; the dissection is brought back onto the wall of the esophagus. The remainder of the esophagectomy is completed by blunt dissection on the esophageal wall.

In cases where the resection is deemed palliative, the entire dissection is performed on the esophageal wall without opening the pleural surfaces or dividing the azygos vein, thoracic duct, and aortic branches under direct vision.

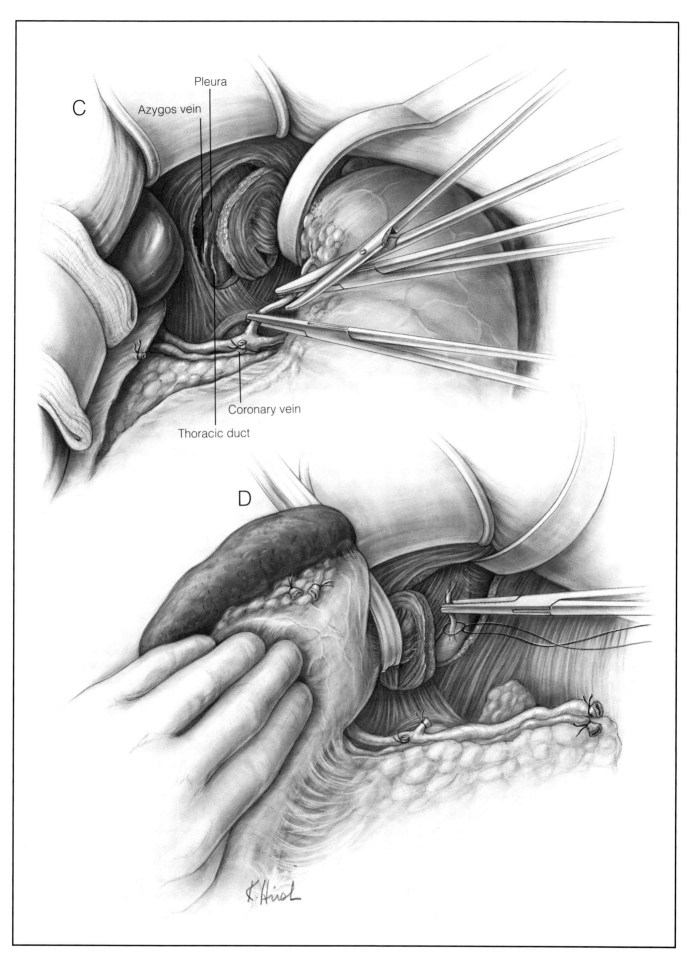

C

Pleura

Azygos vein

Coronary vein

Thoracic duct

D

K.Hirol

With the local resection in the region of the tumor completed, the remainder of the esophagus is dissected bluntly. Through the right cervical incision, the esophagus is removed from the back wall of the trachea. The stay sutures in the strap muscles and thyroid gland provide medial retraction to avoid injury to the recurrent nerve. As the esophagus is encircled, the dissection must stay exactly on the wall of the esophagus to leave both recurrent laryngeal nerves intact.

From below, the surgeon's hand is passed through the widened hiatus, and remaining attachments of the muscular esophageal tube are avulsed right on the wall of the esophagus to leave long stumps of vessels which will go into spasm and retract to provide hemostasis in most cases. When the operator's hand is in the mediastinum, compression of the heart occurs. The anesthesiologist must be alerted to the risk of bradycardia or hypotension. This maneuver with the surgeon's hand must be done intermittently to allow normal heart action between brief periods of dissection.

E

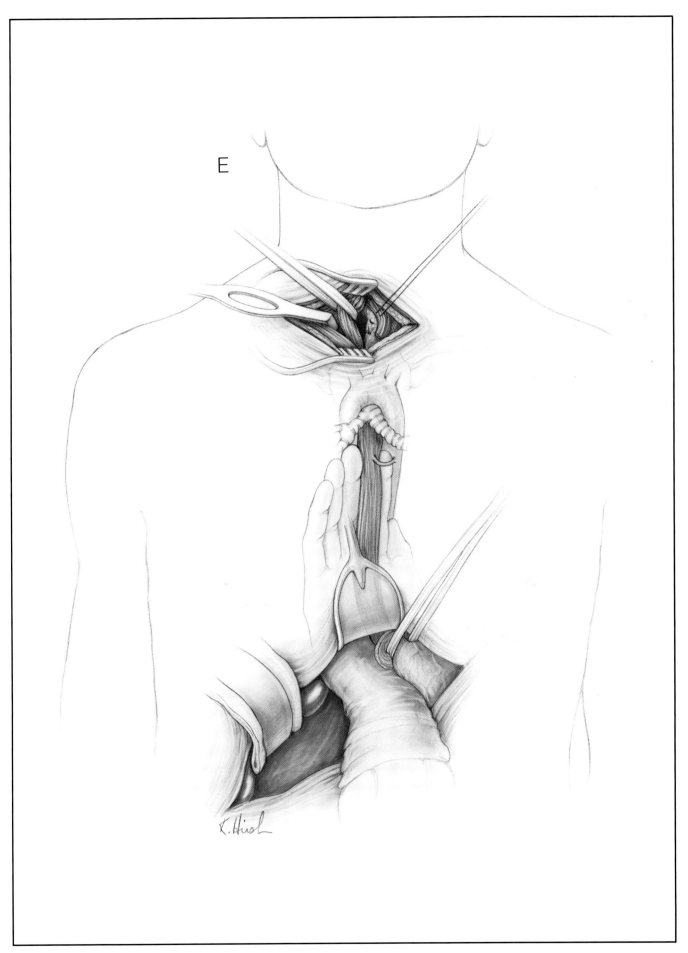

Maneuvers that are helpful in freeing the esophagus from the region of the pulmonary hila, aortic arch, and tracheal bifurcation are shown. The operator's fingers may be inserted through both the cervical and abdominal incisions until they meet in this region, and a circulation motion on the wall of the esophagus facilitates to free the organ at this point where it is bound most tightly. When this is complete, the specimen should now be ready for extraction from the mediastinum.

 The esophagus is removed from the membranous portion of the trachea by blunt dissection near the carina. Proximal to this the surgeon performs sharp scissor dissection on the wall of the trachea under direct vision.

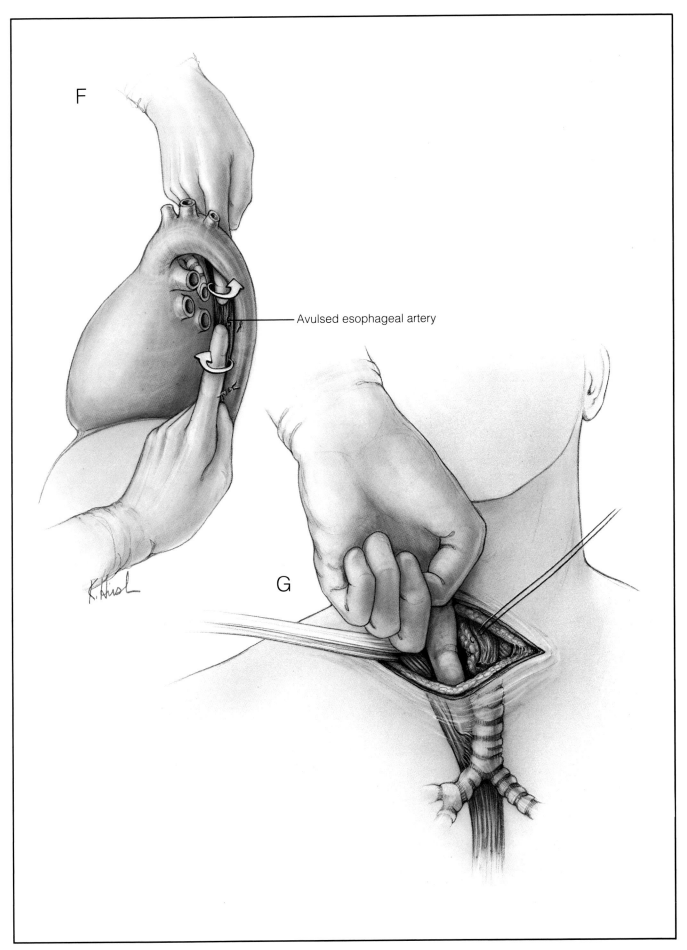

Avulsed esophageal artery

The cervical esophagus is clamped leaving an adequate length for reconstruction by preserving 3 or 4 cm of peristalsing esophagus. The esophagus is extracted from the mediastinum. For this tumor in the intra-abdominal segment of the esophagus, 10 cm margins of stomach on both the greater and lesser curvature are being obtained. The stomach can be divided by stapler or by clamp and suture technique. Even with this much stomach resected, it is frequently possible to advance the remaining stomach to the neck for an esophagogastric anastomosis. This reconstruction is preferred except in those patients with the most favorable tumors in whom long-term survival is assumed. The risks of esophagitis at the esophagogastric anastomosis may be avoided by the use of a colon interposition.

Unless the pyloric channel is patulous to palpation, a pyloromyotomy closed transversely is carried out.

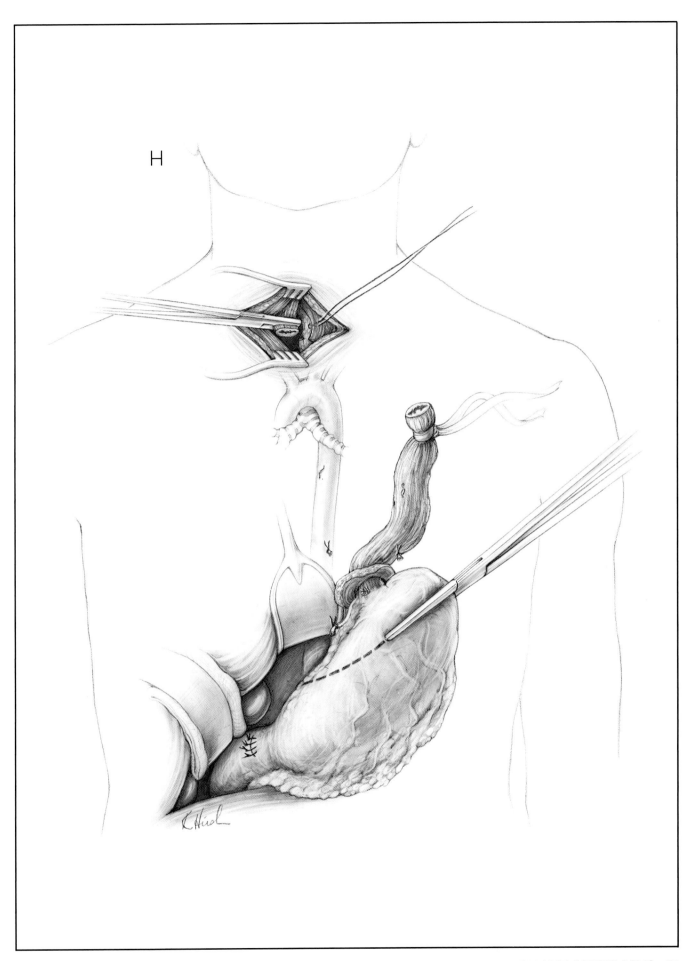

H

# Reconstructions of the Esophagus

Several choices including the whole stomach, gastric tube, isoperistaltic left or right colon, or isoperistaltic jejunum are available for reconstructing the resected esophagus. Suitability of the organ for reconstruction varies among patients so the surgeon should be familiar with several techniques. Operation should be planned with the knowledge that the preferred technique may prove unsuitable, and an alternative must be included in the operative plan.

# 1 | *Reconstruction With the Whole Stomach*

Reconstruction with the whole stomach is illustrated in a patient who has undergone esophagectomy without thoracotomy as illustrated on pages 42 to 51. The incisions are an extended right subcostal and right cervical.

*B*

A point for transection of the stomach is selected 10 cm down the lesser curvature from the tumor in the intra-abdominal esophagus. This generally includes at least three of the descending branches of the left gastric artery. Similarly a point for transection is selected 10 cm from the tumor near the apex of the greater curvature. In this case the spleen is left intact.

After division of all left gastroepiploic arteries, the omentum, previously mobilized from the colon, is resected outside of the right gastroepiploic arcade. The right gastroepiploics are critical in providing blood supply to the interposed stomach. This resection of the omentum is carried down to a point just short of the origin of the right gastroepiploic artery from the pancreaticoduodenal vessel. As indicated by the dotted lines an extensive Kocher maneuver is performed. The hepatic flexure is released from the duodenum. A short pyloromyotomy is made. A long pyloroplasty restricts the advancement of the stomach.

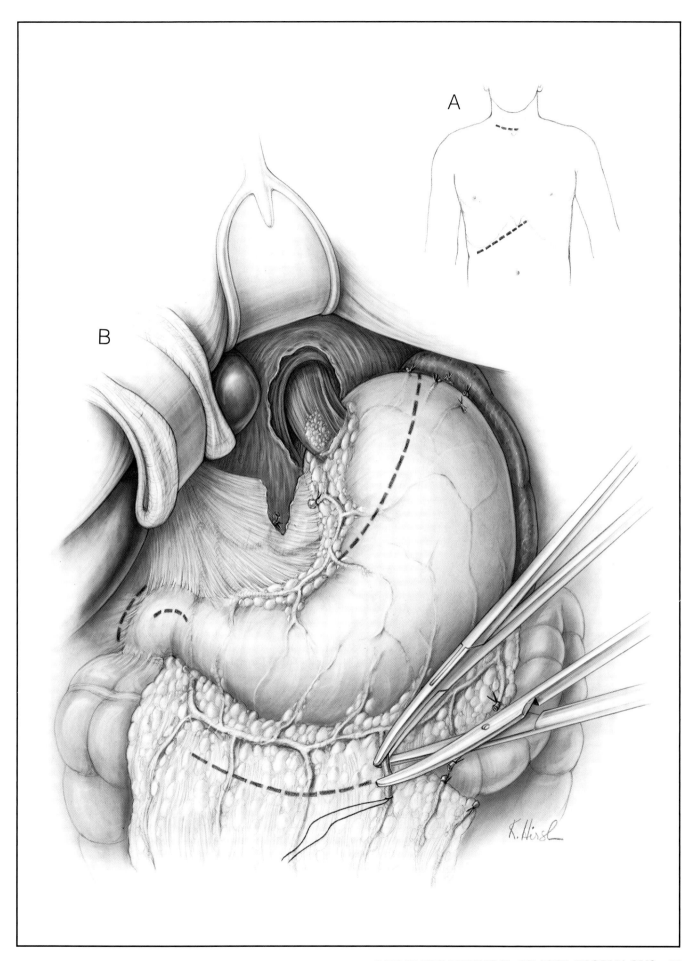

**C** The proximal stomach is resected maintaining the 10 cm margins. This can be done with a stapler or by a hemostatic hand suture over-running a Kocher clamp.

**D** The pyloromyotomy is closed transversely; the elongated lesser curvature is closed; and the apex of the stomach is attached to a malleable retractor which is advanced through the posterior mediastinum and retrieved from the neck.

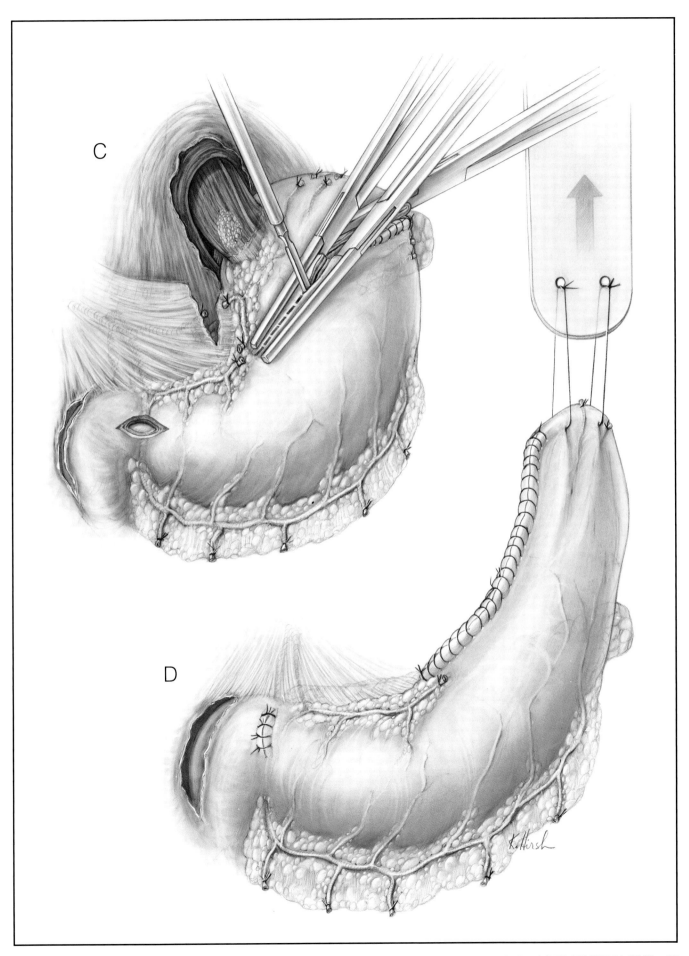

The malleable retractor is retrieved in the cervical incision. The stomach is guided by the surgeon's hand into the posterior mediastinum for advancement to the neck. By using the retractor technique with individual sutures on the greater and lesser curvature aspects, torsion of the stomach in the posterior mediastinum is avoided. After the stomach is in place, the distal antrum or pyloric region is sutured to the margins of the hiatus to prevent herniation of small bowel or colon through the hiatus.

The apex of the stomach is delivered into the cervical incision. The mobilization of the stomach into the neck is facilitated by dividing the strap muscles from the back of the sternum. If this is done, the thoracic inlet is opened significantly, and it is not necessary to resect the head of the clavicle to provide ample space to advance the organ for reconstruction. The apex of the stomach, which is its least vascularized portion, is tacked with several sutures to the prevertebral fascia. The site for anastomosis is identified near the greater curvature of the stomach to avoid a bridge of poorly vascularized tissue between the lesser curvature closure and the site of the anastomosis.

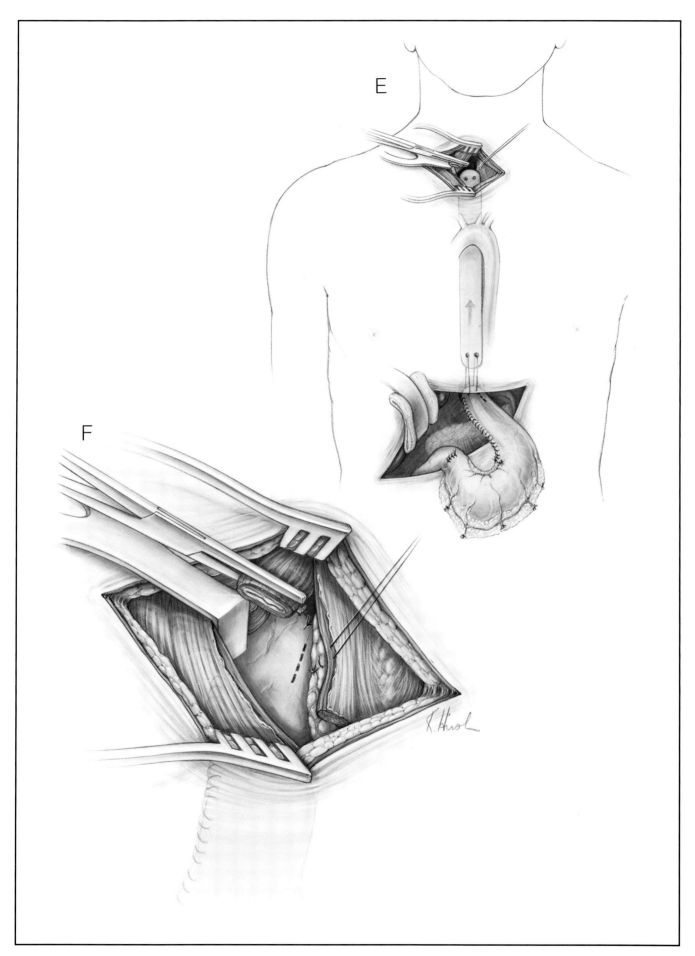

The anastomosis is being performed with a running suture technique. I prefer 5-0 monofilament wire. The details of the anastomotic technique are shown on pages 76 to 79.

The completed whole stomach reconstruction is shown. When whole stomach reconstruction is selected, I perform a pyloromyotomy or pyloroplasty since the pylorus comes to rest in the region of the hiatus and is extremely difficult to expose should gastric retention be demonstrated later and a subsequent pyloroplasty required.

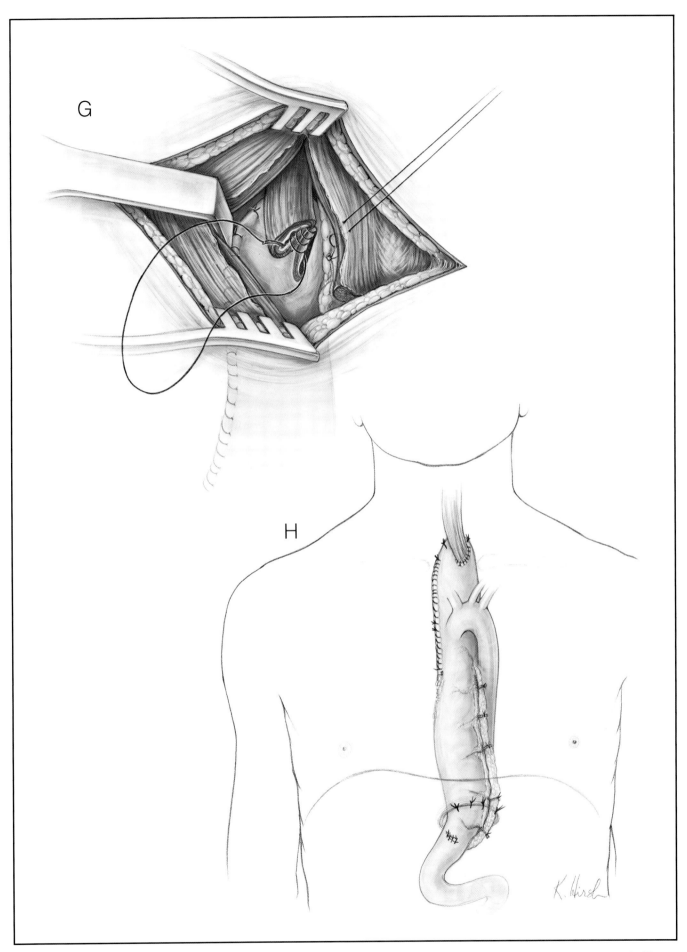

# 2 | *Reconstruction With Isoperistaltic Left Colon*

The use of isoperistaltic left colon for interposition after esophageal resection is preferred for patients with benign disease and those with malignant disease having a good long-term prognosis. The left colon has advantages in avoiding the long-term problem of esophagitis at an esophagogastric anastomosis. The left colon is readily available when the diaphragm is detached through the left thoracotomy approach. The blood supply to the left colon is reliable in 95 percent of patients, and the diameter of the left colon more closely approximates the esophagus. Patients with this reconstruction have been followed more than 20 years in my practice with excellent long-term function.

*A*  In the case illustrated, a short segment interposition is performed following resection of the distal esophagus for benign disease. The left sixth interspace thoracotomy is carried out, and the diaphragm is detached around its periphery.

*B*  The esophagus is divided at the cardia which is closed in two layers. The omentum is mobilized from the mesocolon leaving the gastroepiploic arcades intact on the stomach. For benign disease, the spleen and its gastric attachments are left in place.

*C*  Through the peripheral diaphragm incision the splenic flexure is delivered into the chest. The avascular plane between the omentum and the mesocolon is divided toward the hepatic flexure to improve mobility of the colon. The omentum is resected. The descending colon is mobilized by scissor dissection down the left paracolic gutter to the base of the sigmoid colon mesentery.

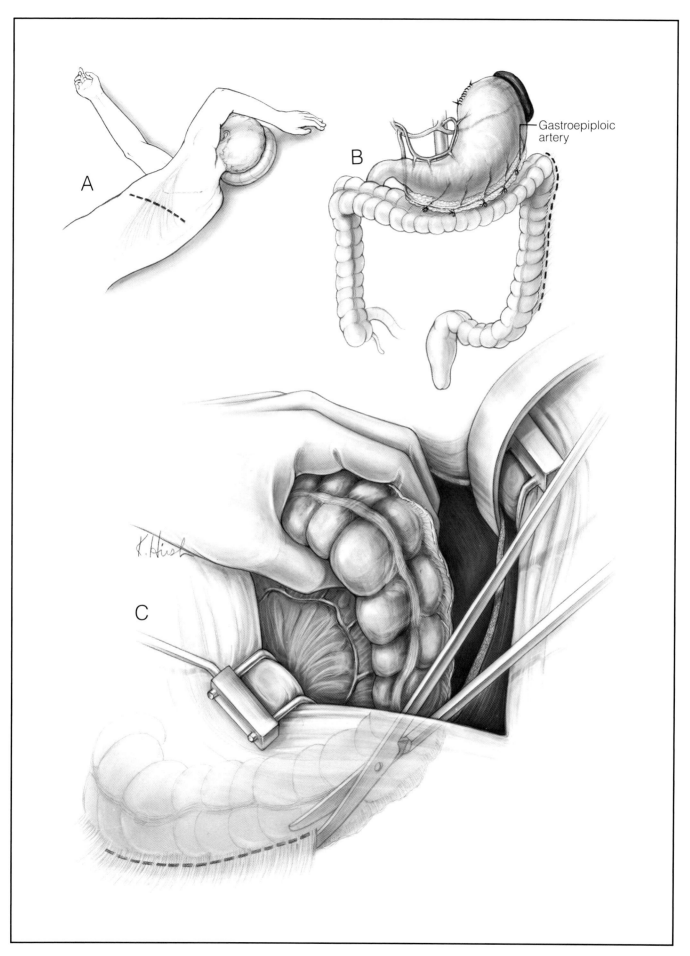

Gastroepiploic
artery

A

B

C

**D** In this patient a short segment interposition is needed to reach below the aortic arch. A portion of the descending colon and the left transverse colon provide the desired length which is measured with a tape. The point for transection of the descending colon is identified and the colon divided with cautery between clamps. Only those vessels immediately adjacent to the colon require division. Often two branches of the left colic artery or a left colic artery and left branch of the midcolic artery can be identified and preserved to the interposed segment.

**E** In this case the point for transection of the transverse colon is identified at point B. Should a long segment interposition to reach the neck be required, the point of transection would be at C. In this case the arcade between the main midcolic and left colic vessels is divided, and the incision in the mesocolon carries down near the base of the mesocolon. The points of division of the vessels for a long or short segment interposition are shown schematically. Occasionally for a long segment, the midcolic artery must be divided near its origin and the marginal artery is divided in the arcade between the mid- and right colic vessels. Transverse cuts in the avascular mesocolon add length to the pedicle by reducing the tethering effect of the mesocolon. MC, midcolic artery; SMA, superior mesenteric artery; IMA, inferior mesenteric artery; MA, marginal artery; LC, left colic artery; AB, ascending branch.

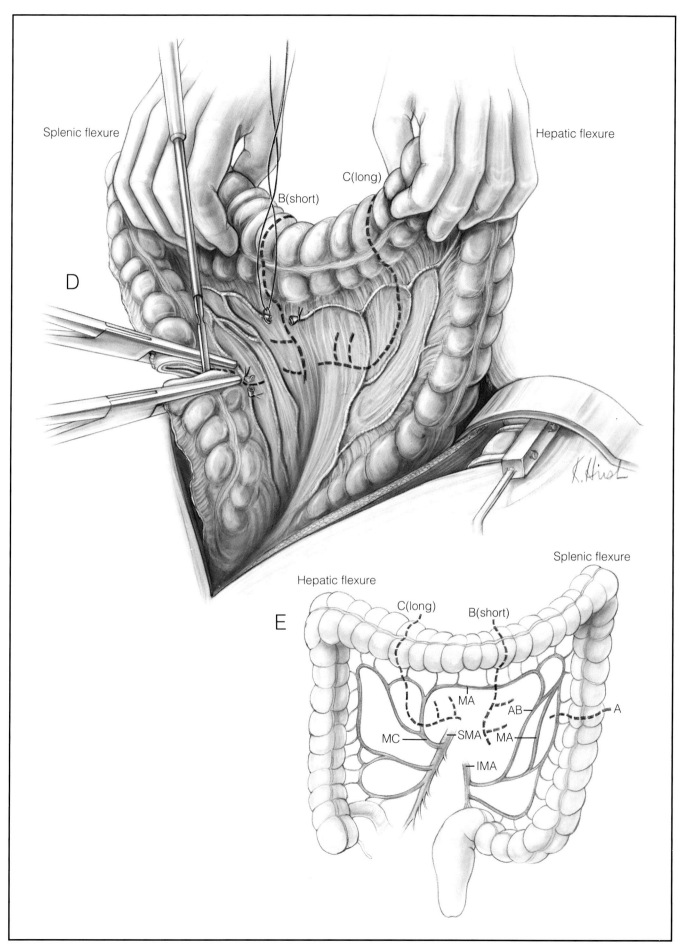

F The colon is divided between clamps. The segment is mobilized and passed behind the stomach into the hiatus. The proximal transverse colon end is advanced into the mediastinum. The remaining right transverse colon is readily mobilized to reach the descending colon for anastomosis avoiding a large incision in the descending colon mesentery and thereby preserving the maximal number of arcades to the splenic flexure.

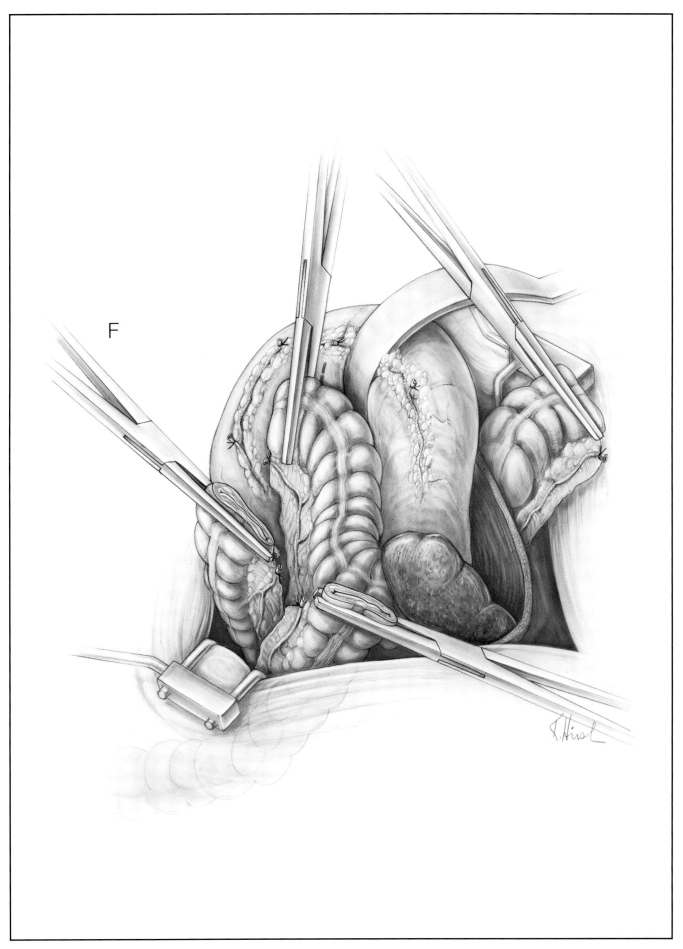

F

While the interposed segment is laying in its new bed to ascertain that the circulation is adequate, the colocolic anastomosis is done. The clamped ends of the bowel are cut away so that the sutures are placed in uncrushed tissue. Plugs of block Gelfoam are placed in the lumen of the bowel in each direction to eliminate spillage. This avoids the need for the application of clamps to the colon, which may danger the microcirculation. The anastomosis is done with a single layer running technique preferably with 5-0 monofilament wire. In all patients in whom a colon interposition may be employed, a mechanical bowel prep is used preoperatively with nonabsorbable antibiotics given the night before surgery.

The colocolic anastomosis is completed. The point for performance of the cologastric anastomosis selected approximately one-third of the way down the stomach from the fundus on the posterior wall near the greater curvature. Two stay sutures are placed in the stomach near the gastroepiploic arcade, and an incision is made from the greater towards the lesser curvature. The cologastric anastomosis is started at the base of this incision with running sutures carried up both sides of the anastomosis. An open anastomosis is done. The tissue included in the Kocher clamp is excised.

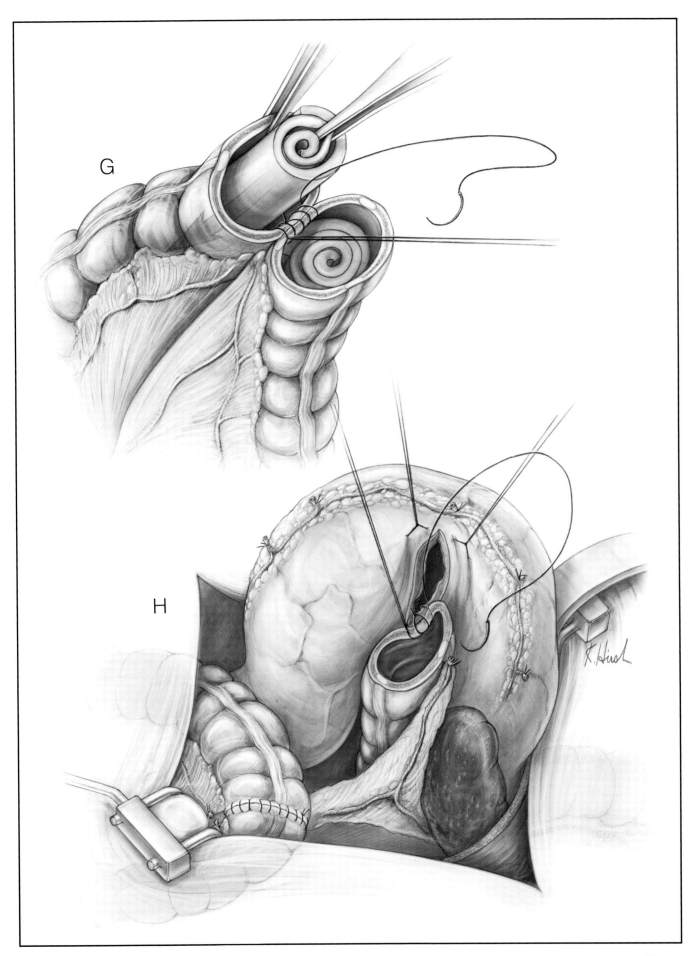

G

H

K. Hirsch

*I* The esophagocolic anastomosis is done just below the aortic arch in this short segment interposition. After completion of the anastomosis the colon is pulled down manually under some tension to avoid redundancy and anchored at the margins of the hiatus with interrupted sutures.

*J* The completed interposition is shown. The remaining gastric fundus is reattached to the diaphragm in front of the hiatus in a horseshoe fashion. This prevents access of small bowel or colon to herniate into the hiatus and also provides a partial fundoplication around the intra-abdominal segment of colon.

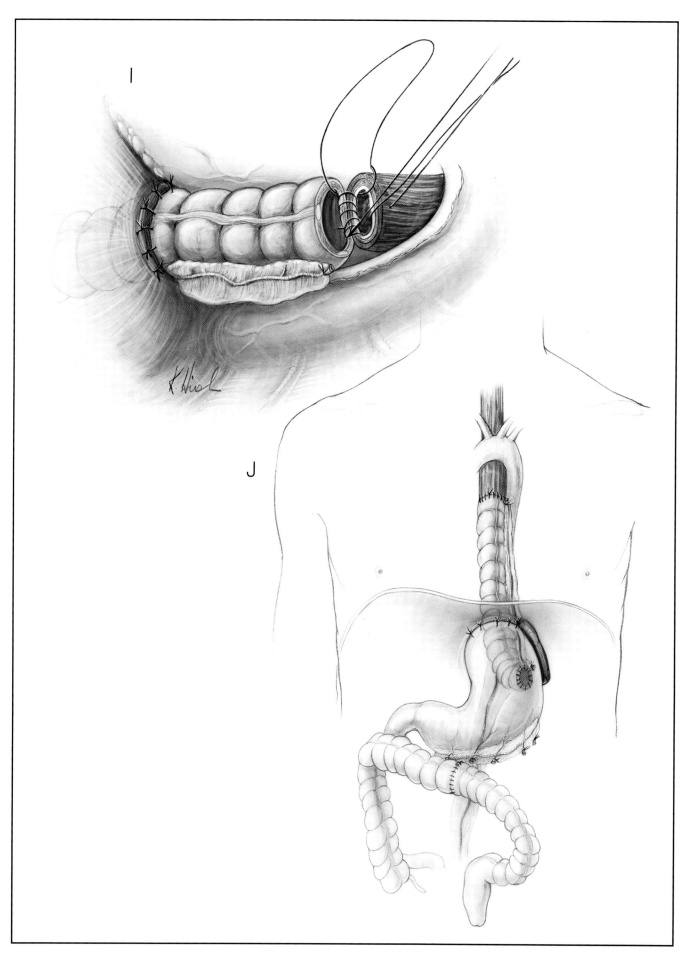

# 3 | *Long Segment Interposition*

When the entire intrathoracic esophagus is to be replaced by colon through a left thoracotomy, the bowel is divided at point C on page 65. This means dividing the midcolic artery near its origin and including the midcolic arcades in continuity with the left colic arcade to provide the extra length desired.

*A* The colon is mobilized as illustrated in the preceding section with the additional length acquired by division of the midcolic artery. The esophagus is previously mobilized below the aorta for resection as in a case of a Barrett's esophagus extending to or above the aortic arch. The dissection is carried under the aortic arch and a new incision made in the pleura proximal to the aortic arch and posterior to the left subclavian artery. The esophagus is encircled at this point and transected. The specimen is removed. Stay sutures are placed on the mesenteric and antimesenteric borders of the colon.

*B* Using a curved Semb clamp the stay sutures are grasped beneath the aortic arch. The colon is advanced taking care not to rotate the clamp and interposition. The stump of the esophagus is closed with three mattress sutures to which the needles are left attached.

*C* The needles from the mattress sutures are subsequently used to attach the stump of the colon segment to the closed esophagus. Sufficient colon is mobilized to reach easily to the neck which can be palpated from within the thorax. With the colon held at this level, the bowel is straightened out and attached to the margins of the hiatus before closing the thoracotomy.

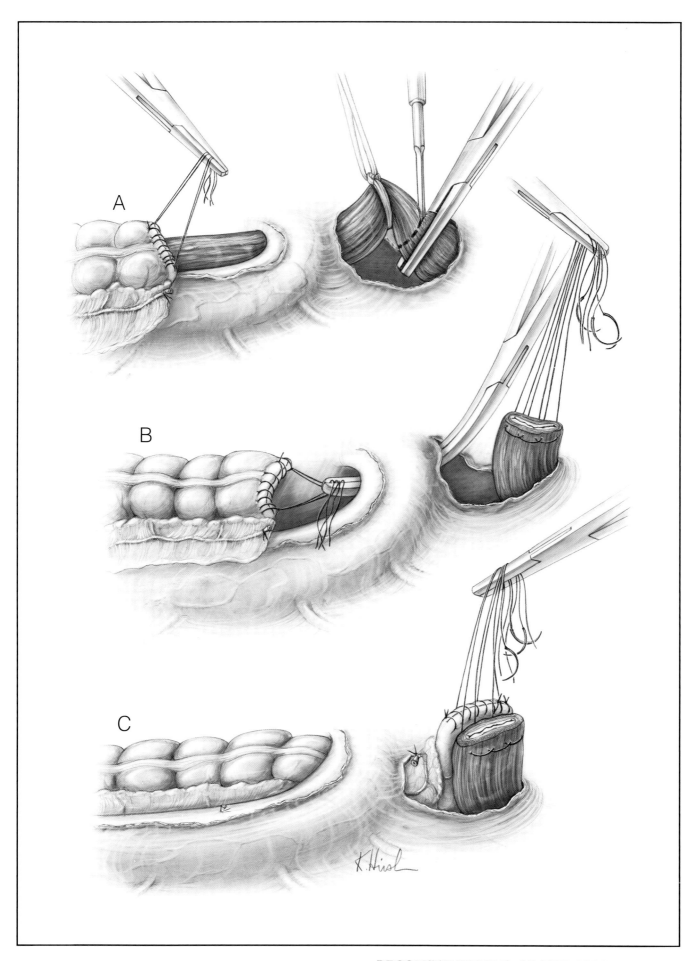

The final anastomosis of the long segment colon is made to the esophagus in the neck through a left cervical incision. The final reconstruction is illustrated.

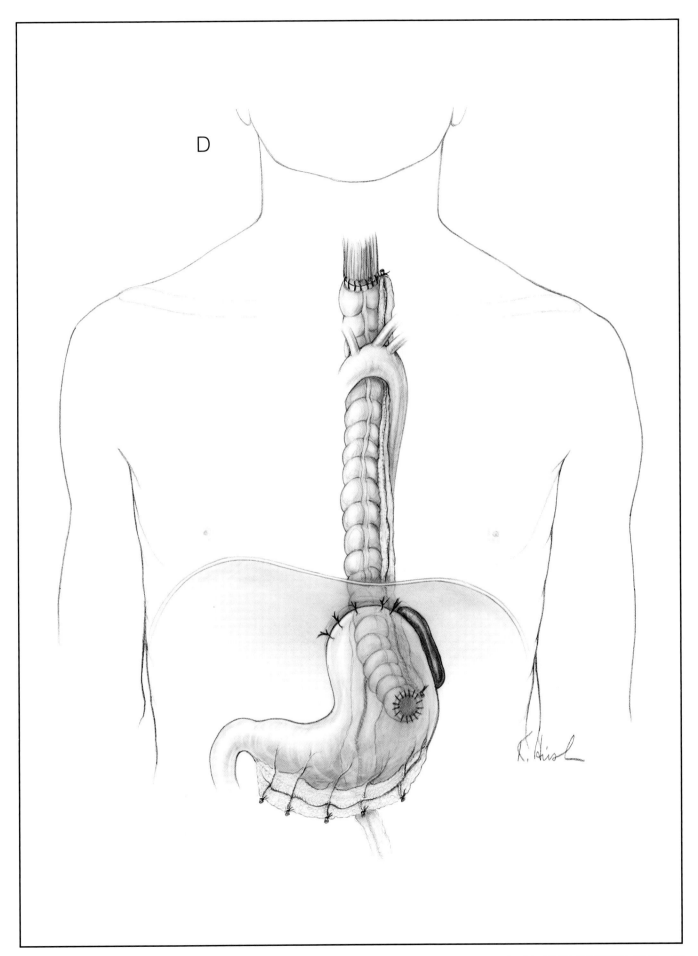

D

# 4 | Anastomotic Techniques

A variety of one, two, and three layer sutured or stapled esophageal anastomoses are described. Recognizing that the esophagus, unlike other parts of the digestive tract, has only one layer, the submucosa, containing collagen and elastic tissue to hold sutures, a single layer anastomosis is preferred. While a stapled anastomosis can be performed with a leakage rate comparable to hand sewn anastomosis (i.e., about 5 percent), stapled anastomoses have a higher reported stricture rate, presumably because of the turned in cuff of tissue. This is avoided by a single layer hand sewn anastomosis. Using the illustrated single layer interrupted or running technique with 5-0 monofilament wire, an anastomotic leakage rate at all levels in the esophagus of 6 percent and a stricture rate requiring dilatation of less than 2 percent has been maintained for over 20 years.

*A* The techniques described illustrate anastomosis of the colon to the esophagus end-to-end, but the same methods are used for a jejunal or gastric anastomosis to the esophagus. For an interrupted anastomosis, an initial stitch is placed posteriorly with a single square knot in the 5-0 wire suture placed within the lumen. The sutures pass somewhat obliquely through the wall of the colon so that a larger bite of serosa than mucosa is taken. This creates a slight inversion. Since only the submucosal layer of the esophagus has the strength to hold sutures, a through and through stitch is placed at a generous distance back from the cut end. The esophageal mucosa tends to retract so it must be carefully viewed as each stitch is placed. Sutures are always passed from inside to out on the esophagus so the needle can be seen to catch a good bit of mucosa.

*B* Traction sutures may be placed in the esophagus under slight tension to maintain full diameter of the esophageal lumen. The interrupted sutures are continued across the back wall and up the side away from the surgeon.

*C* When all but the last two or three stitches have been placed, the final sutures are made with the knots tied on the outside.

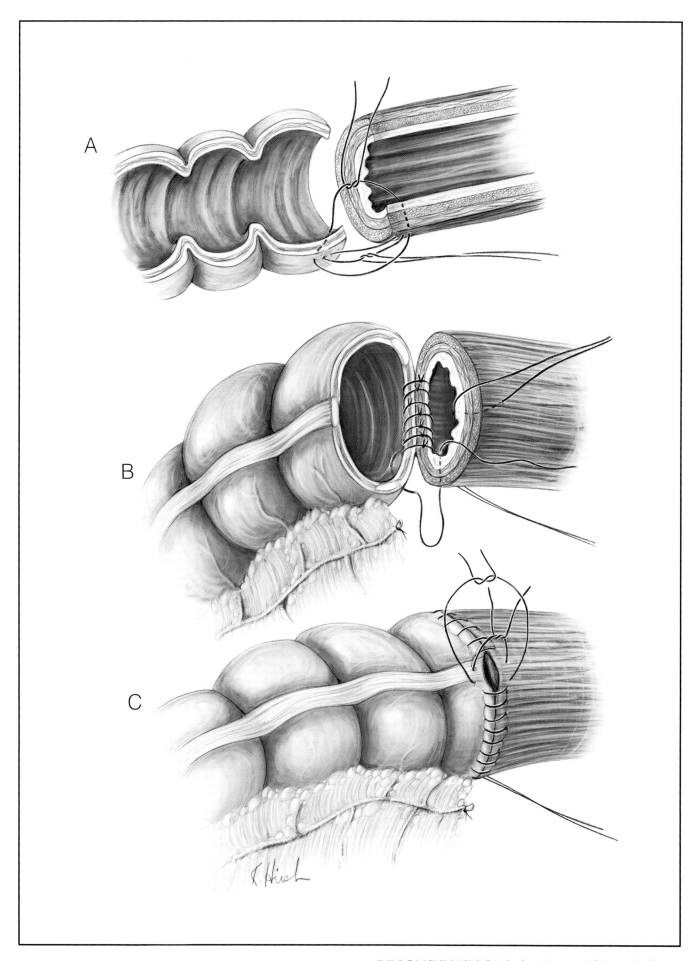

# 5 | *Continuous Suture Anastomotic Technique*

A running 5-0 wire anastomosis is my usual preference.

**A** A single anchoring seromuscular suture is placed posteriorly away from the cut edge to begin the aposition of the divided ends.

**B** The running suture passes first from inside to outside on the wall of the esophagus to be certain that a substantial piece of mucosa and submucosa is included in the bite. The suture is continued from the outside to inside on the colon taking a larger amount of serosa than mucosa.

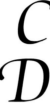

**C** **D** When the anastomosis is nearly complete, the sutures are brought back to the outside of the colon and esophagus. The anastomosis is completed with a Connell suture passing from outside to inside and reversing back to outside on either side of the final gap. The two ends are tied. After completion of the anastomosis, the circumference is carefully inspected for any gaps between the running sutures. If such gaps are found, an interrupted Lambert stitch is placed into the superficial layers to turn in the defect.

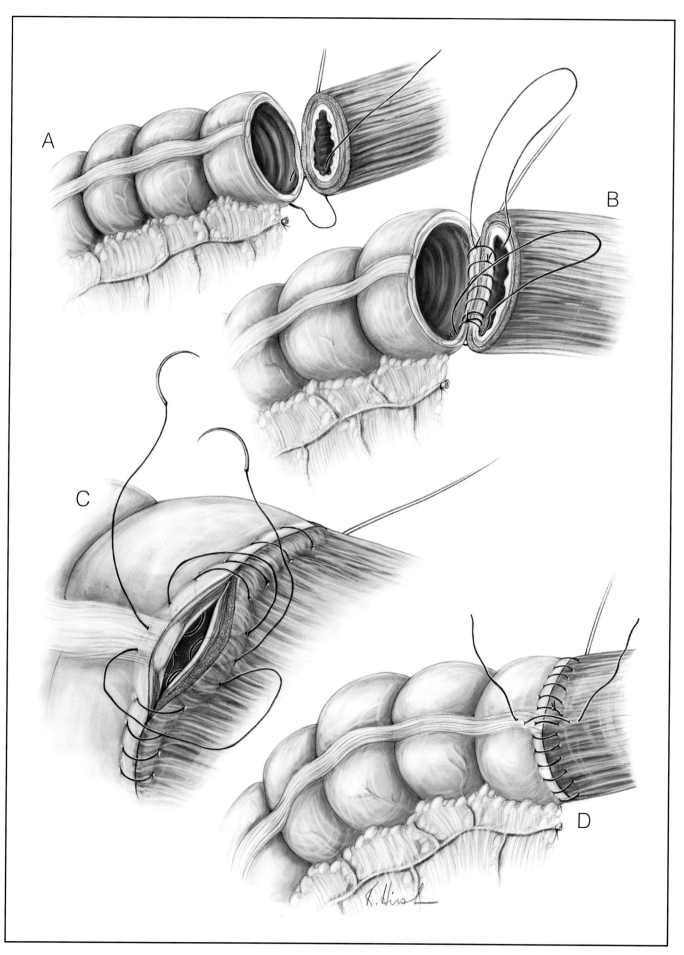

# 6 | *Jejunal Interposition*

A jejunal interposition to reconstruct the esophagus is especially appropriate where a short segment of esophagus is resected for benign disease. Because of the variability and shortening of the mesentery, the jejunum is rarely suitable for a long segment interposition.

*A* In the case illustrated, a resection is being performed for a benign esophageal stenosis following previous procedures. An upper midline incision is made and extended below the umbilicus to provide better exposure to the small bowel mesentery.

*B* The jejunal segment is based in this patient on a distal branch of the mesentery artery with proximal arteries being divided. Transillumination of the mesentery aids in planning the vessels to be divided. The initial point of transection is selected one or two arcades away from the ligament of Treitz. In this case the first and second branches from the superior mesenteric artery are left intact with division of the arcade between the two portions of the second branch. The third mesenteric artery branch is divided near its origin, and the interposition is based on the fourth branch from the superior mesenteric artery. The arcade between the fourth and fifth branches are divided near the distal point of bowel transection (B-B'). Nontraumatic Potts vascular clamps are applied to each vessel before it is divided to be certain that there is a distal pulse in each case.

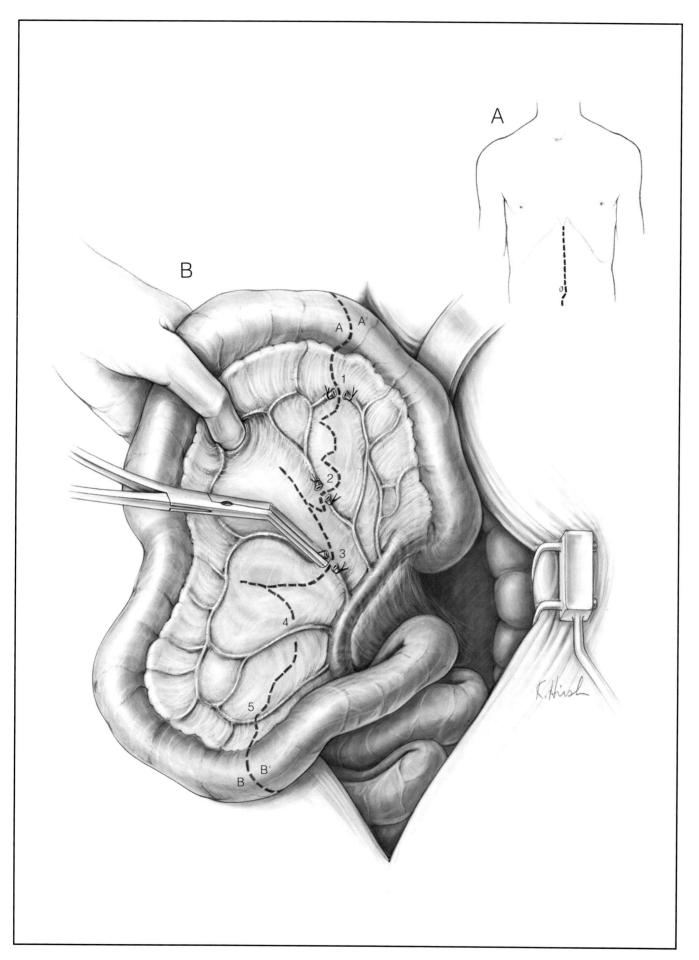

*C* The jejunal segment is mobilized for advancement behind the stomach based on the fourth mesenteric artery. Several incisions are made in the mesentery between vessels to allow the pedicle to elongate. The proximal and distal jejunum at points A′ and B′ are anastomosed end-to-end using a single layer technique. A wide gap in the mesentery is left open because it is less likely to cause small bowel obstruction than if the surgeon attempted to close the defect leaving a small hole at the root of the mesentery.

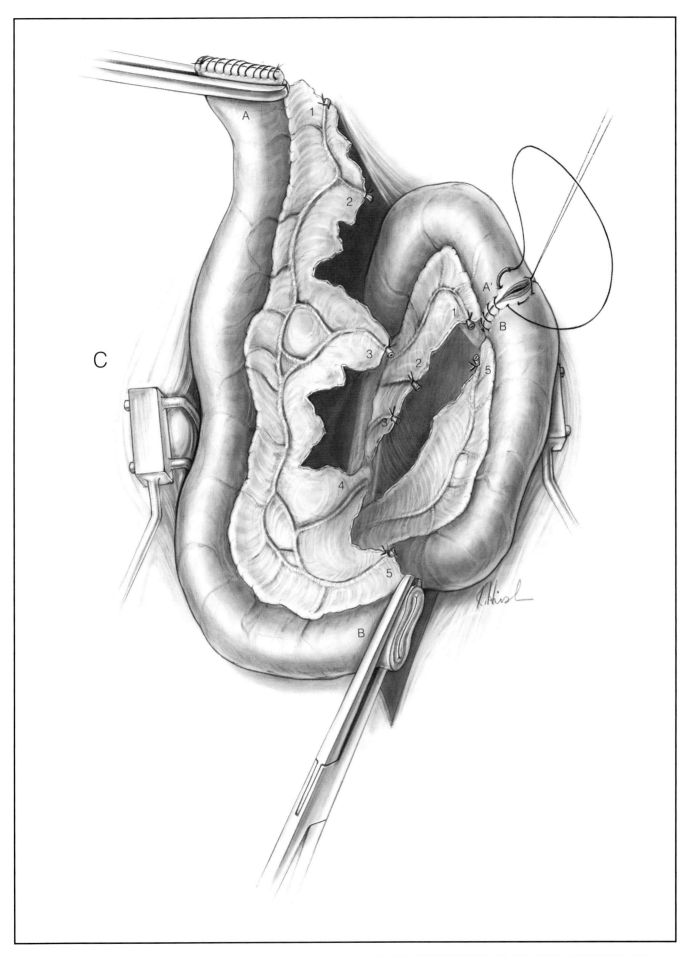

C

An incision is made in the transverse mesocolon to the left or right of the midcolic artery depending on how the pedicle lies best. The distal esophagus has been mobilized within the hiatus and the stomach reflected superiorly. The proximal jejunum (point A) is brought up behind the stomach. The end is oversewn and tacked loosely to the esophagus in the posterior mediastinum.

The distal end of the interposed segment (point B) is also passed through the mesocolon. An anastomosis is made to the stomach near the greater curvature approximately one-third of the way down from the fundus. The abdomen may now be closed.

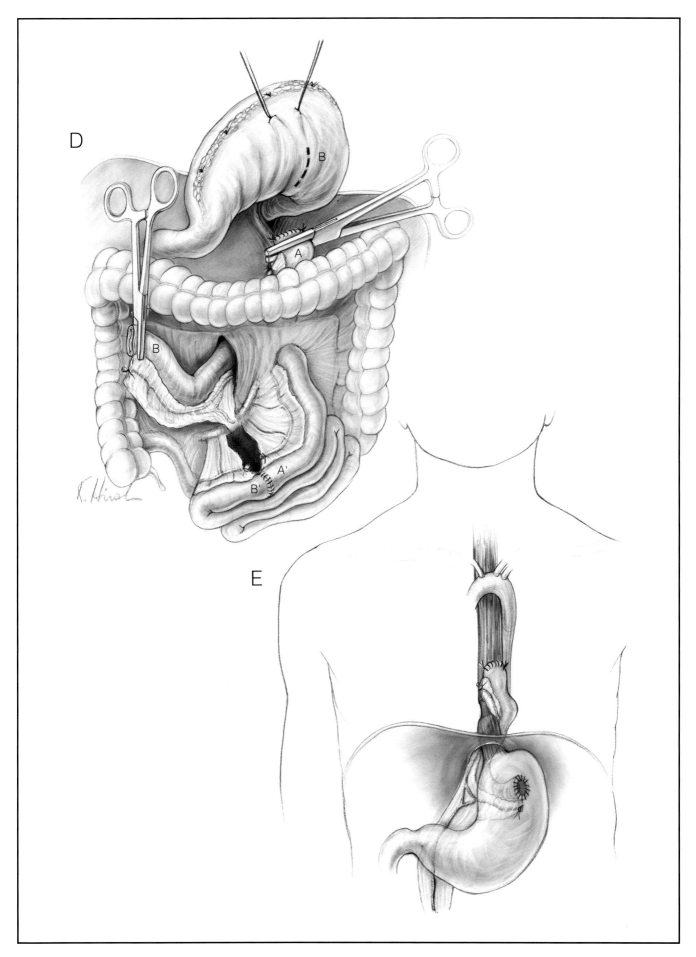

**F** The esophageal resection and esophagojejunal anastomosis are made through a left thoracotomy in the sixth interspace.

**G** The proximal jejunal segment having been previously passed through the hiatus is now brought up into the chest behind the esophagus. The localized segment of esophagus containing the stricture is mobilized. The cardia is divided with care being taken that all squamous epithelium is included within the esophageal specimen so that the closure is done in gastric epithelium to avoid ulceration.

**H** The cardia is closed in two layers, the first for hemostasis over the resecting clamp and the second to turn in the defect. The point for transection of the esophagus above the stenosis is identified.

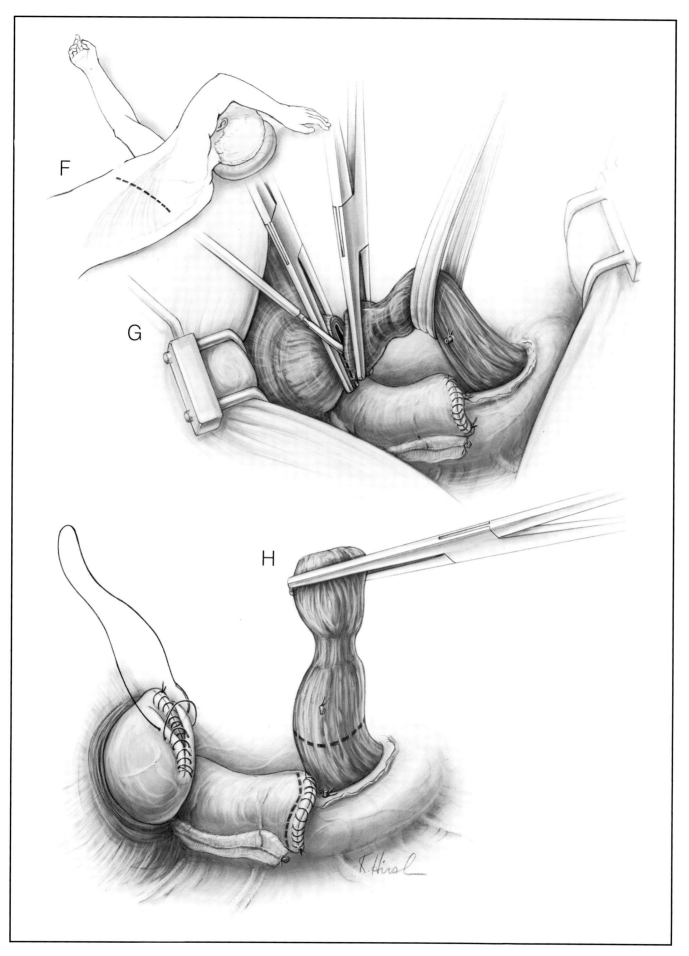

F

G

H

*I*   The anastomosis is begun between the freshly divided esophagus and open end of the jejunum, the previously closed end of the jejunum having been amputated. A running suture technique is employed passing each stitch first from inside to outside through the esophagus and ending inside the jejunal lumen. Because the hiatus is enlarged during the dissection by passage of the jejunum alongside the esophagus, one or more sutures are placed in the esophageal hiatus posteriorly.

*J*   After the anastomosis is complete, the jejunum is pulled downward so that the intrathoracic segment is straight. Several sutures are placed anterolaterally between the margins of the hiatus and the jejunum to fix it in this location and prevent herniation along side the interposed segment.

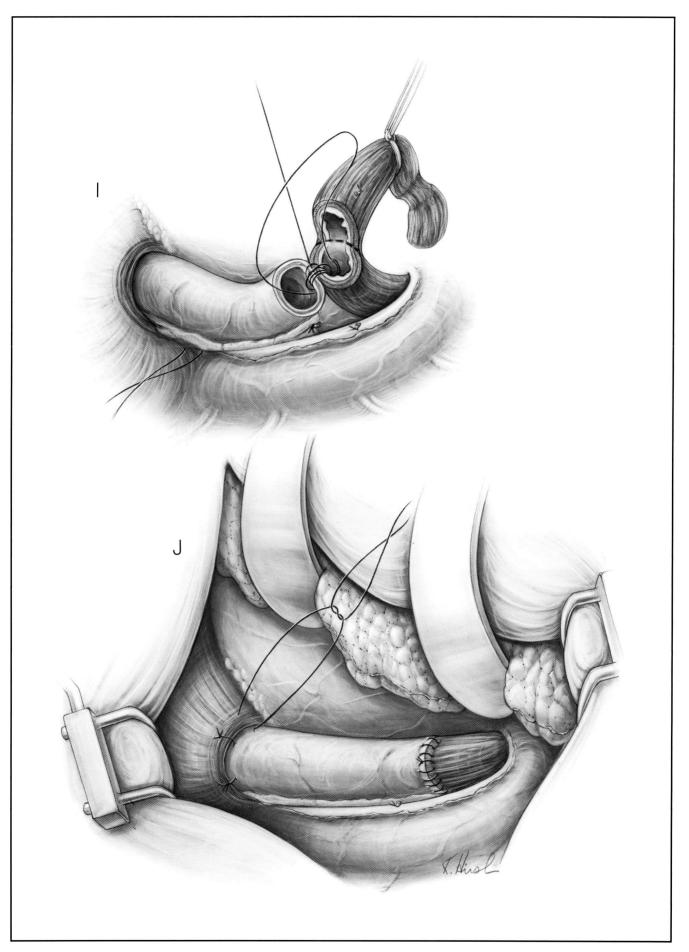

# 7 | *Gastric Tube Interposition*

A reversed gastric tube reconstruction is favored for esophageal replacement by some surgeons. There are several disadvantages to this technique that have not made me enthusiastic for its use. These include the reduction in capacity of the residual stomach, the long staple and suture lines required to fashion the tube, and the potential for irregular tube dilatation if the tube is not fashioned with uniform diameter. In patients with this reconstruction whom we have studied, gastric secretion persists in the tube so the complication of esophagitis at the esophagogastric anastomosis is not totally eliminated.

*A* Preparation of the gastric tube is done transabdominally, usually through a midline or extended right subcostal incision. After the esophagus is prepared for transection, usually for benign disease, an incision is made just proximal to the pylorus where the right gastroepiploic artery is divided.

*B* A large bougie (size 50 F or greater) is placed retrograde through this opening along the greater curvature. A stapler is positioned with several applications with the greater curvature wrapped around the bougie. This tube should not be made too snugly over the bougie since it is necessary to turn in a second layer to reinforce the staple line. Care must be taken to preserve the splenic vessels and left gastroepiploic arcade which serves as the blood supply to the tube. This operation should not be done if the spleen has been removed.

*C* The gastric tube closure is reinforced with a running layer of suture to turn in the staple line. This runs the entire length of the tube and remainder of the greater curvature. The bougie is left in place as a stent to prevent undue narrowing while this is accomplished. It is especially important that the junction of the tube with the residual stomach not be narrowed. When the tube is completed, it can be passed through the hiatus into the mediastinum for anastomosis with the esophagus as illustrated previously for the colon and jejunal interpositions.

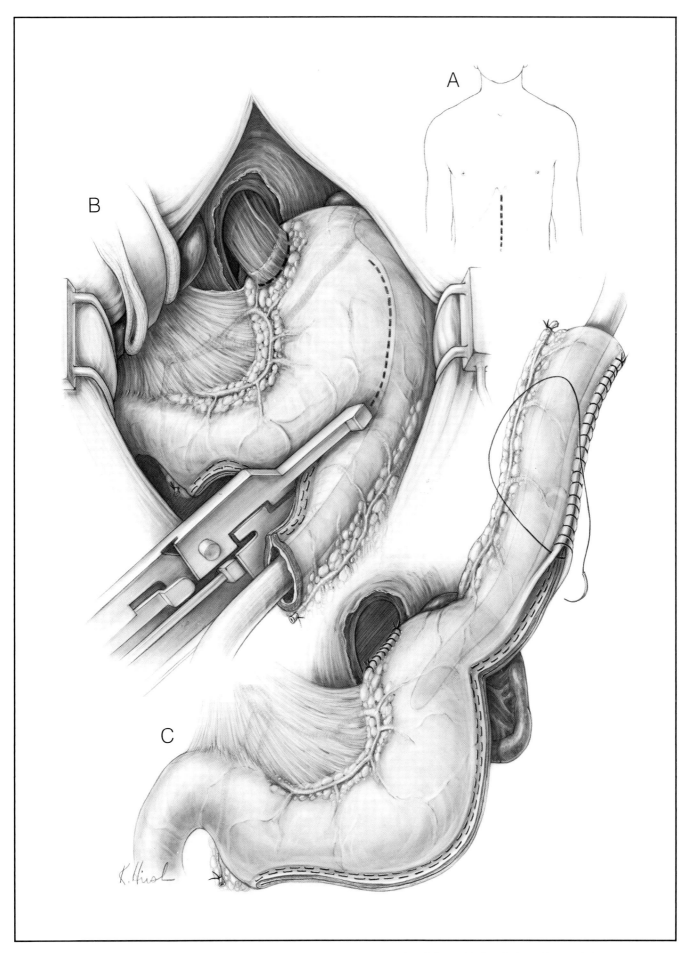

# 8 | *Reconstructions After Total Gastrectomy: Jejunal Loop*

For carcinomas extending from the proximal stomach into the distal esophagus or visa-versa, a total gastrectomy and distal esophagectomy may be the resection of choice. If enough esophagus can be mobilized to be drawn down through the hiatus for anastomosis, a jejunal loop reconstruction is preferred. When more esophagus must be resected to achieve a satisfactory margin proximal to the tumor a colon interposition between the esophagus and duodenum is the reconstruction of choice.

When total gastrectomy and distal esophagectomy are performed entirely through a midline abdominal incision, exposure is ideal for the jejunal pouch interposition. The self-retaining "upper hand" retractor is used.

After the stomach and distal esophagus are resected, the duodenum is closed. A segment of jejunum is prepared distal to the first arcade approximately 10 cm from the ligament of Treitz.

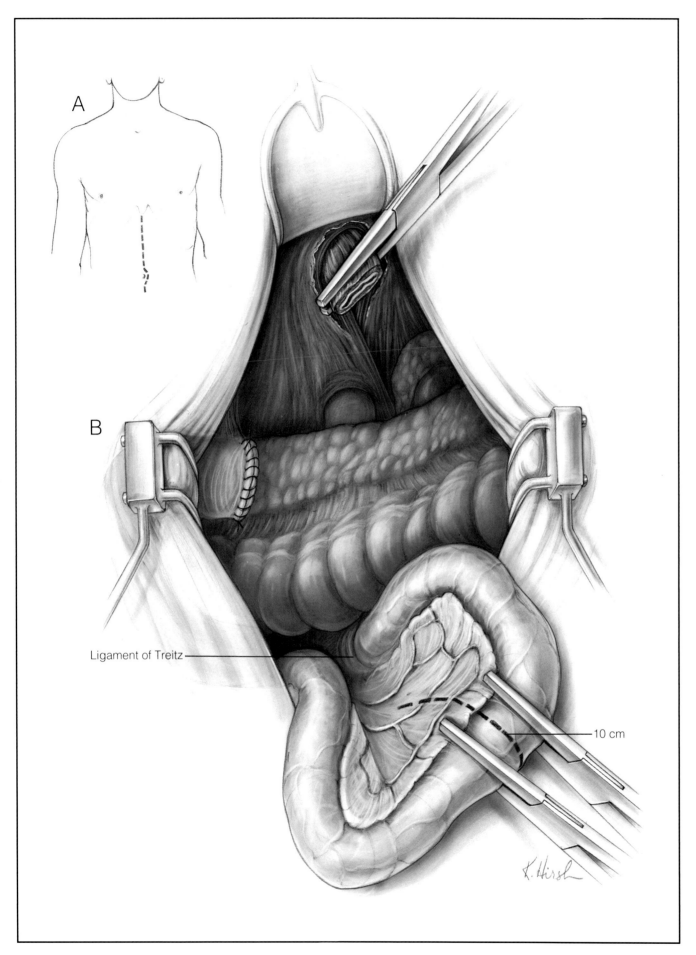

Ligament of Treitz

10 cm

**C**

To provide some digestive capacity, I prefer to prepare the jejunal interposition as a B loop (Lygadakis). The jejunal loop is folded back on itself so that the afferent limb is approximately 15 cm long. Five centimeters from the apex a side-to-side anastomosis of approximately 3 cm long is made between the afferent and efferent loop. Again a single layer anastomosis is performed to keep the lumen as wide as possible.

The end of the afferent loop is anastomosed end-to-side into the efferent loop approximately 5 cm further down the bowel. The esophagogastric anastomosis is made at the apex of the loop on its anterior wall. The jejunum can be folded over the anastomosis to reinforce the single layer suture line. Finally, the proximal jejunum coming from the ligament of Treitz is anastomosed to the distal jejunum at least 40 cm distal to the lowest anastomosis of the reconstructed pouch.

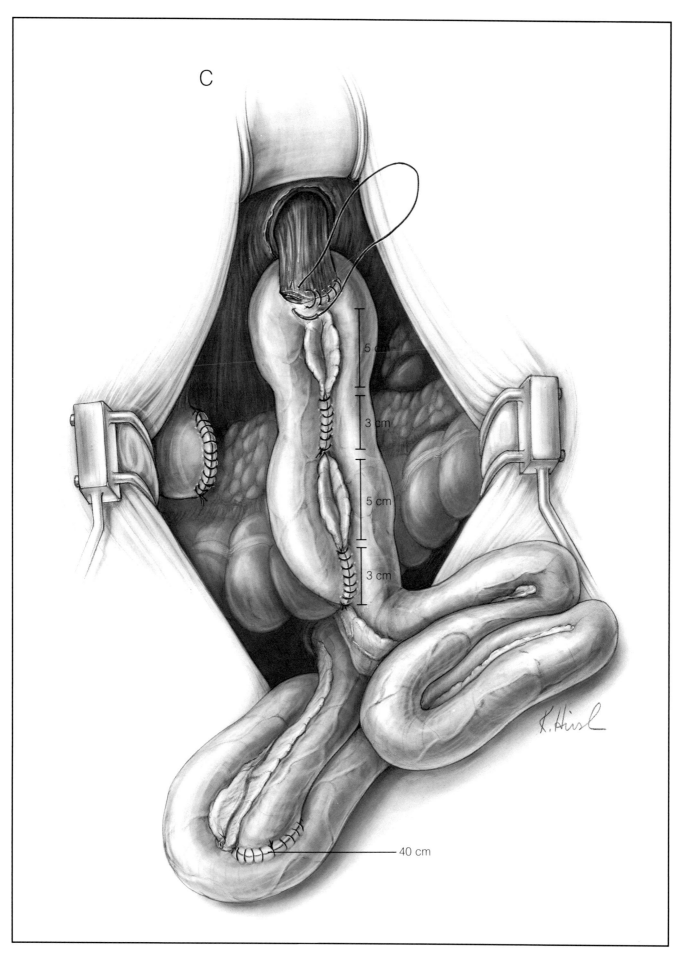

C

5 cm

3 cm

5 cm

3 cm

40 cm

# 9 | Reconstructions After Total Gastrectomy: Isoperistaltic Left Colon

**A** When an adenocarcinoma of the cardia is approached through a left thoracotomy and found to be arising from the stomach, a total gastrectomy in addition to distal esophagectomy may be performed. This can be readily accomplished through the left sixth interspace thoracotomy with the diaphragm detached around its periphery.

**B** The left and transverse colon are mobilized as described on pages 62 to 75. Either a long or short segment colon interposition can be used depending on the amount of esophagus to be resected. The colon is passed in the usual way through the hiatus with an end-to-end anastomosis made to the esophagus at the point selected for transection. The distal segment of the colon is anastomosed end-to-end into the duodenum. The colon is pulled distally under some tension to avoid intrathoracic redundancy, and it is anchored in the hiatus to fix it in a straight position and to avoid herniation into the chest. Because of the capacity of the colon, this reconstruction offers some pouch effect to aid in the digestive process. For this reason, a longer segment of colon is better functionally than a short segment which may permit duodenal esophageal reflux and offer a limited capacity of the pouch.

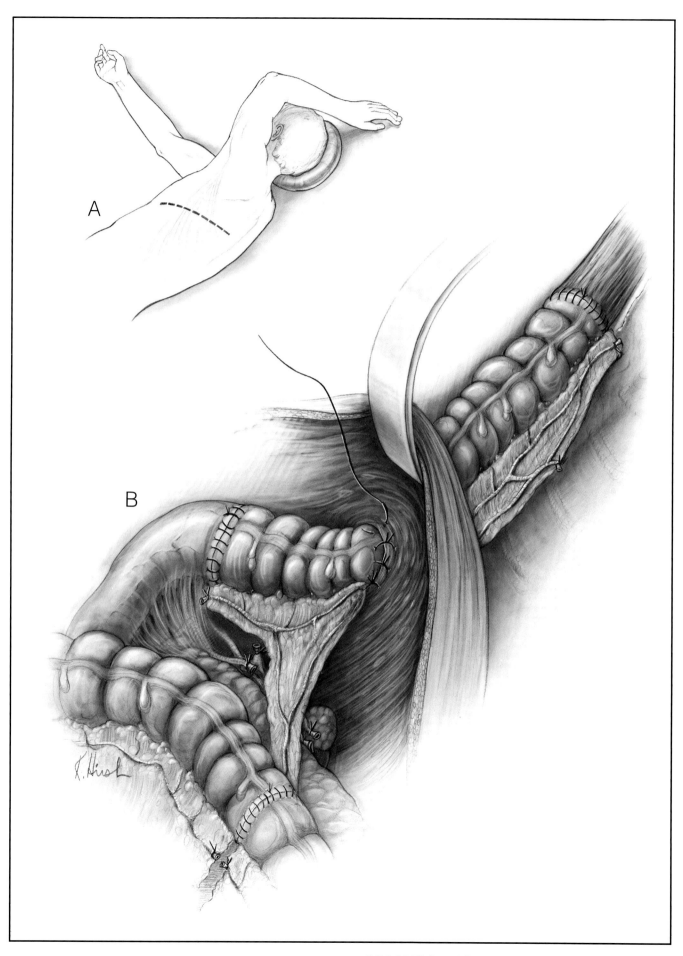

# Bypass Procedures

In patients such as those with a tracheoesophageal fistula, previous esophagectomy without reconstruction, or some instances of lye stricture, it may be decided to do a reconstruction by bypass without concurrent esophagectomy. This may be accomplished transthoracicly, but more commonly substernally, and rarely subcutaneously.

# 1 | *Substernal Left Colon Bypass*

*A*

The procedure is carried out through an abdominal, preferably extended right subcostal, incision and a cervical incision centered on the midline.

*B*

The substernal tunnel is started by making an incision behind the xiphoid leaving a cuff of diaphragm attached to the xiphoid for fixation of the interposed organ.

*C*

The situation where the esophagectomy has been carried out through a right thoracotomy with the chest closed is illustrated. The abdomen is open, and preparations are made for the substernal bypass. It is important to close the hiatus with interrupted permanent sutures to avoid a herniation into the chest. The cardia is closed on the gastric side. Using a retractor on the abdominal wall alongside the xiphoid process, a 4-cm incision is made through the diaphragm muscle by cautery. It may be necessary to dissect the diaphragm away from the pericardium, which can be identified by palpation as the muscular incision is deepened.

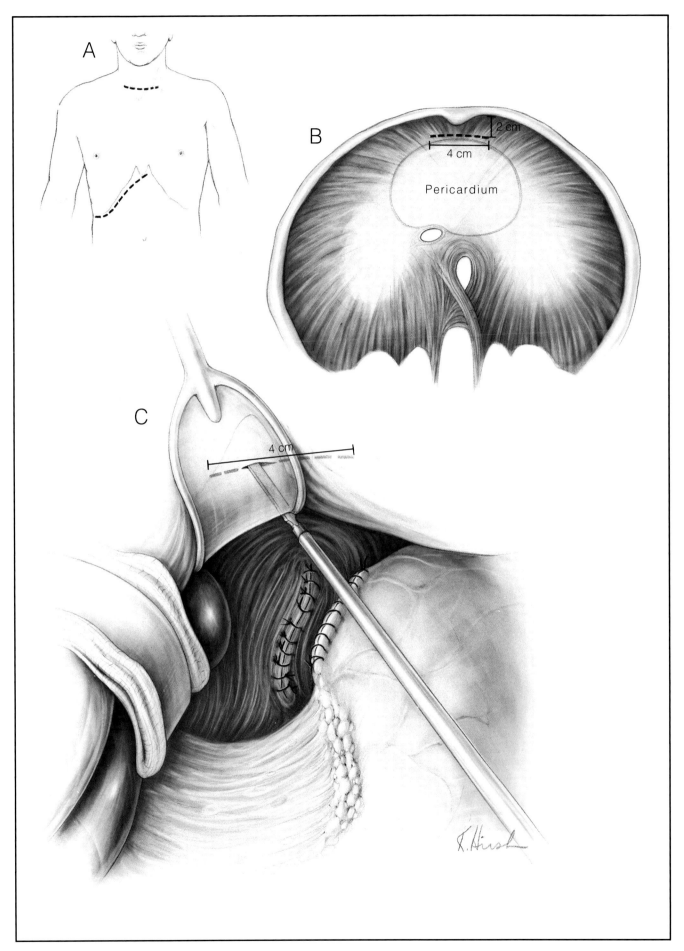

A transverse cervical incision is made 1 cm above the sternal notch, and flaps are elevated. To provide free access to the retrosternal region, the sternal insertions of both strap muscles are divided with cautery. In some instances it is helpful to divide the sternal head of the sterno-cleidomastoid muscle as well. This provides adequate space in the thoracic inlet to advance the interposed organ without resection of clavicular heads or manubrium.

Using blunt finger dissection from above and below, the substernal tunnel is created. The pleural reflections in front of the pericardium are pushed laterally in an effort to avoid opening the pleural cavity on either side. A long malleable retractor is placed through the substernal tunnel to confirm its patency.

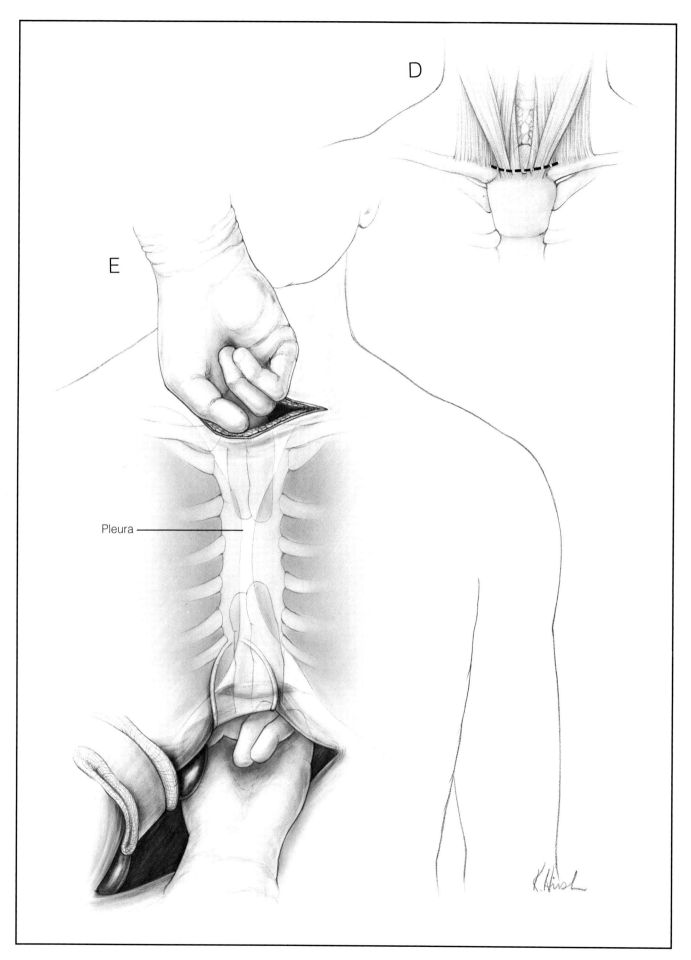

D

E

Pleura

*F*   To reach the neck a long segment colon interposition is prepared based on the ascending branches of the left colic artery. The midcolic artery is divided near its origin to preserve its communicating arcades. Counter incisions in the avascular mesocolon are made to achieve length.

*G*   After the colon segment for interposition is isolated, it is passed behind the stomach. The cologastric anastomosis is made near the greater curvature approximately one-third of the way down from the gastric fundus. The proximal colon is closed with sutures left long on the mesenteric and antimesenteric border. These sutures are attached to the malleable retractor which is passed through the substernal tunnel and functions as a "sled" to advance the colon through the tunnel to the neck.

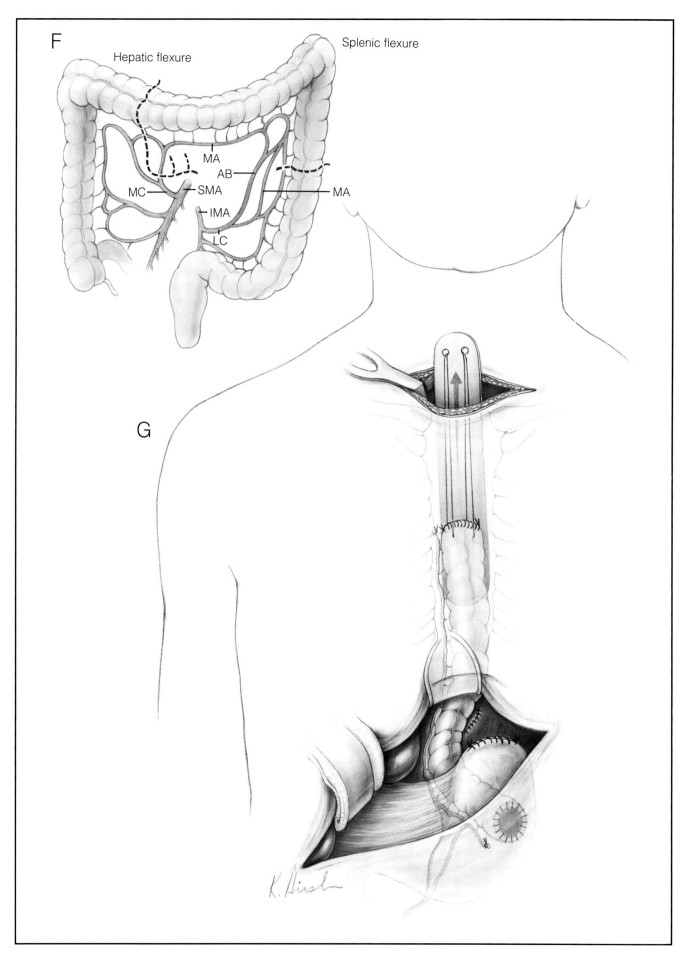

An end-to-end anastomosis is made to the esophagus in the neck. It is important to leave several centimeters of peristalsing esophagus below the cricopharyngeal sphincter to prevent regurgitation from the colon back into the hypopharynx. After the interposition is in place, it is pulled downward under gentle traction and sutured with interrupted stitches to the margins of the opening in the diaphragm. This is done to avoid herniation of small bowel and to prevent the colon from becoming redundant within the thorax.

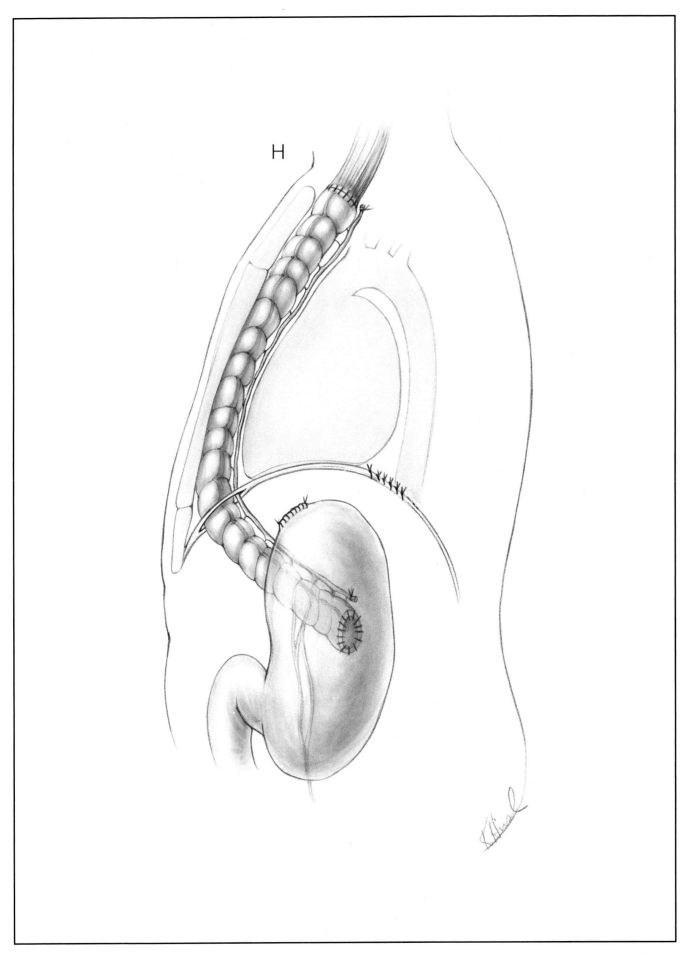

H

# 2 | *Substernal Stomach Bypass*

When the colon is not suitable for the bypass, the whole stomach may be used in a substernal position. The stomach is preferred when several centimeters of peristalsing esophagus cannot be preserved. The stomach is less likely than the colon to have retrograde peristalsis leading to regurgitation into the pharynx in the absence of a peristalsing esophageal barrier.

The stomach is mobilized as for reconstruction with the whole stomach (see pages 54 to 61). Since the pylorus may end up in the subxiphoid location or within the substernal tunnel, a pyloromyotomy or pyloroplasty is performed routinely as access to this area may be difficult subsequently. If the esophagus is left in situ and the stomach is used for the bypass, the esophagus should be drained to prevent a closed chamber in the posterior mediastinum. This may necessitate drainage to a roux-en-y jejunal loop (not illustrated).

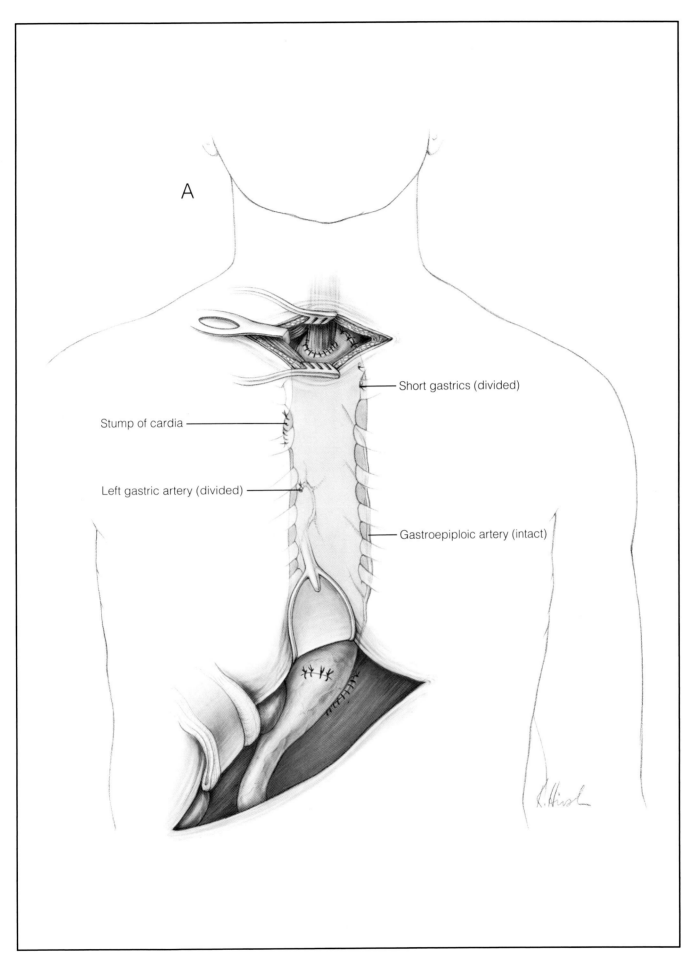

A

Short gastrics (divided)

Stump of cardia

Left gastric artery (divided)

Gastroepiploic artery (intact)

# 3 | *Subcutaneous Right Colon Bypass*

The use of the right colon and ileum for a bypass is illustrated. When the right colon and ileum are used for esophageal reconstruction through any location, they are mobilized in the same fashion as illustrated here for a subcutaneous bypass.

*A*

Several incisions, including a cervical incision which may be extended downward as a T to facilitate delivery of the colon, a cutaneous incision in the right inframammary fold to assist in tunnel construction, a right subcostal incision made only through the fascia layers from within and not through the skin as the site of exit for the colon, and a midline laparotomy for mobilization of the colon, are necessary for a subcutaneous bypass. Recently, we have employed tissue expanders in conjunction with our plastic surgery team to create this subcutaneous tunnel from the neck to the costal margin. These devices are put in place at least 2 weeks before the planned subcutaneous interposition. They create an excellent fibrous lined tunnel through which the colon can be easily advanced.

*B*

The steps in creating the tunnel are illustrated. After the midline laparotomy is carried out and the colon mobilized, an incision is made slightly below the right costal margin from within the abdomen to the subcutaneous space passing through peritoneum, transversalis fascia, and the muscle layers lateral to the rectus muscle. With blunt dissection, a tunnel is made from this site of exit from the abdomen to the inframammary skin incision. Again, with blunt dissection the inframammary incision is connected to the right cervical incision. Advance implantation of tissue expanders along this course is most helpful.

The points for division of the transverse colon, mesocolon, ileum, and mesentery are shown. The interposition is isoperistaltic and based on the midcolic artery. The right colic and ileal colic vessels are divided with care taken to be certain that the arcades are intact. Approximately 20 percent of patients do not have continuity of the arcades across the ileocecal valve. This limits the length of the segment to the right transverse and ascending colon. This may or may not provide sufficient length to reach the neck. Counter incisions are made in the avascular portions of the mesentery to provide additional length. An appendectomy is routinely performed.

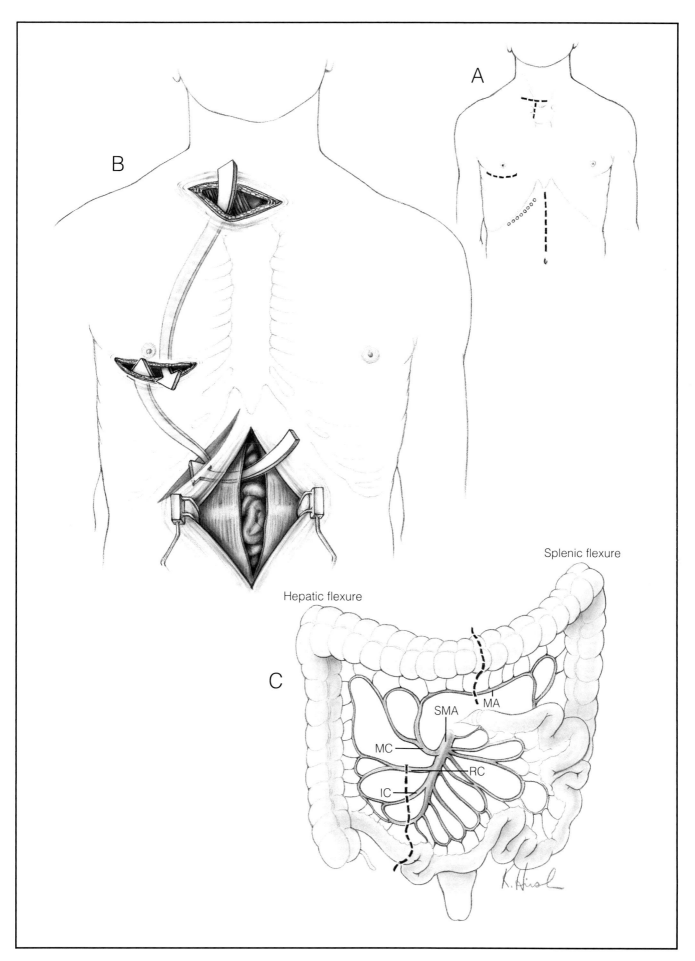

Hepatic flexure

Splenic flexure

SMA

MC

RC

IC

MA

The isoperistaltic segment is passed up through the previously constructed tunnel. If required for adequate length, the terminal ileum may be anastomosed to the esophagus. However, if there is sufficient length, it is preferable to amputate the cecum and terminal ileum and make the anastomosis to the ascending colon. The ileocecal valve is the narrowest point in the digestive tract, and use of the ileum prevents some patients from eating solid food which will not pass readily through the ileocecal valve. Occasionally, a side-to-side opening of the ileocecal valve into the cecum may be necessary.

After all anastomoses are complete, the transverse colon is sutured to the margins of the abdominal wall counter incision to prevent herniation upward into the tunnel. Skin incisions are closed as is the midline laparotomy incision. The residual terminal ileum is anastomosed end-to-side to the midtransverse colon.

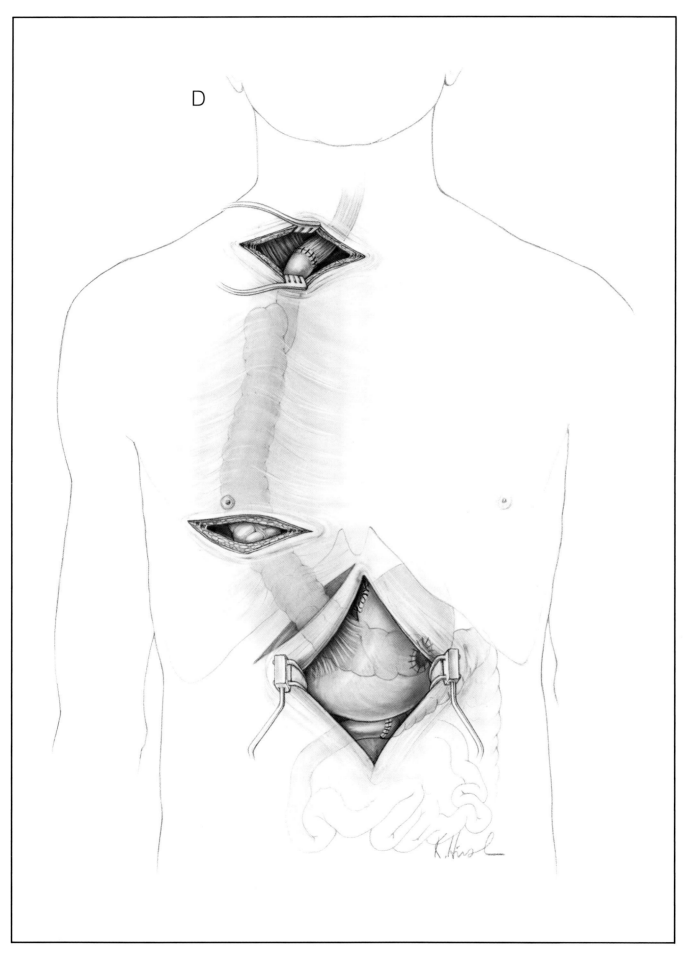

D

# Antireflux Repairs

Several antireflux repairs have been introduced over the past 35 years that incorporate similar principles for control of reflux. These repairs are known by the names of their developer although modifications may be introduced. The repairs are presented as those done through a thoracotomy, the Belsey or Nissen operations, and those done through a laparotomy, the Nissen, Hill, and Guarner procedures. Each of these repairs has stood the test of time and has proved to control reflux long-term in 85 to 90 percent of cases. There are specific indications for using a thoracic or an abdominal approach, so the surgeon treating reflux disease should be familiar with either approach.

# 1 | Transthoracic Antireflux Repairs: Belsey Mark IV Operation

*A*

The distal esophagus and hiatal hernia are approached through a left thoracotomy performed in the sixth intercostal interspace as described on pages 6 to 11.

*B*

The esophagus is mobilized from the mediastinum up to the level of the aortic arch. Care is taken to leave the right sided pleura intact. After full mobilization, tension is applied to the esophagus by the encircling tape. An incision is made through the phrenoesophageal membrane at a right angle to the gastroesophageal junction.

*C*

To enter the peritoneal cavity, the scissors must cut through the pleura into the thoracic fascia blending with the intra-abdominal fascia to create the phrenoesophageal membrane, retroperitoneal fat, and peritoneum. Continued upward tension on the esophagus draws these layers up through the hiatus where they can be incised.

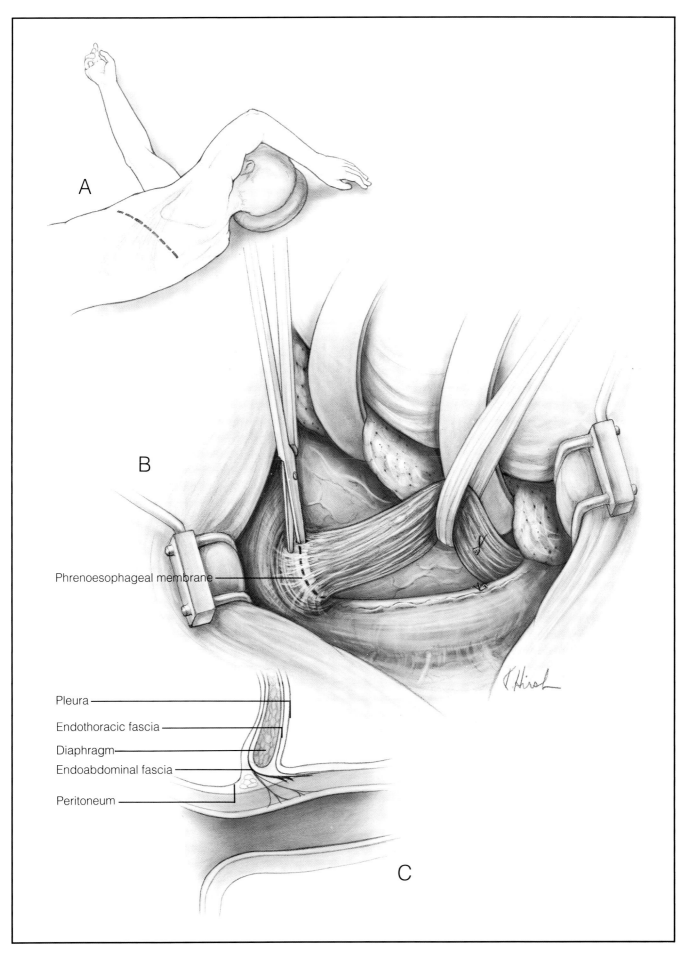

A

B

Phrenoesophageal membrane

Pleura
Endothoracic fascia
Diaphragm
Endoabdominal fascia
Peritoneum

C

Repositioning of the distal esophagus beneath the diaphragm is a critical component of an antireflux repair. The gastroesophageal junction must be fully mobilized in the hiatus. The dotted lines indicate the incision into the greater and lesser peritoneal sac. Coming off the cardia laterally and medially, the vagus nerves pass through the phrenoesophageal membrane at the locations of the upper edge of the greater and lesser omentum. Blood supply to the cardia is adjacent to the nerves with a branch of the left gastric artery anterior and adjacent to the right vagus nerve and the branch of the left anterior phrenic artery just anterior to the left vagus nerve.

 The greater peritoneal cavity is opened by incising the phrenoesophageal membrane circumferentially from one vagus nerve to the other. The arterial branches are ligated as they are encountered. A branch of the inferior phrenic artery communicating with the left gastric system crosses on the posterior aspect of the hiatus. Belsey has stressed the importance of dividing this artery to provide hemostasis as the lesser sac is entered.

 The stomach is delivered anteriorly and access to the greater peritoneal sac is complete. The posterior tissue in the decussation of the crus is pulled up, and clamps are applied to the fold of the phrenoesophageal membrane and peritoneum to secure the communicating artery. Scissor incision between these clamps provides access to the lesser sac and completes the mobilization.

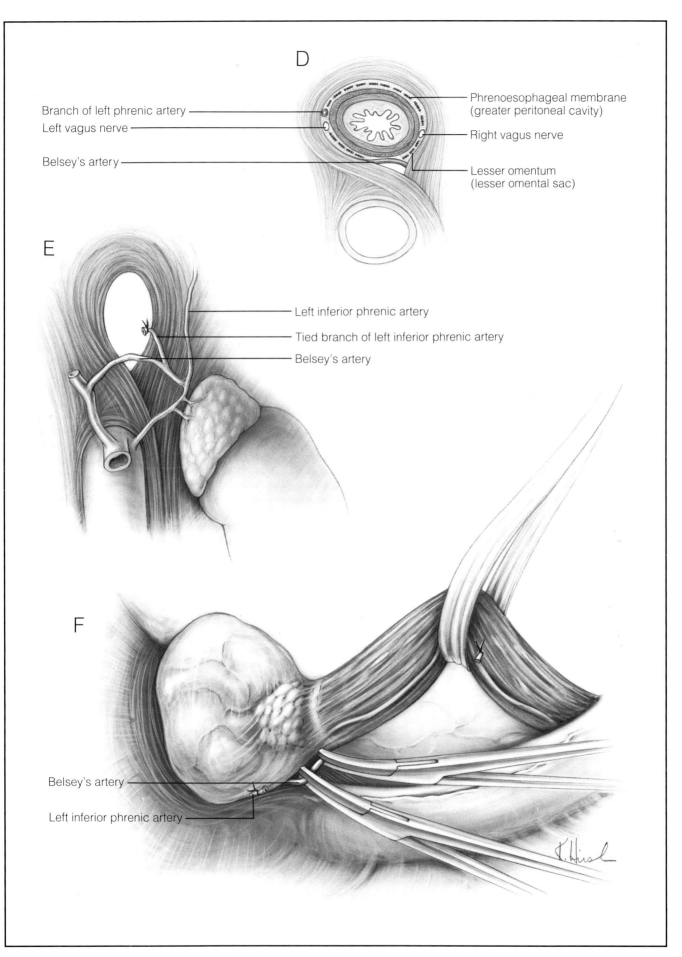

D

Branch of left phrenic artery

Left vagus nerve

Belsey's artery

Phrenoesophageal membrane
(greater peritoneal cavity)

Right vagus nerve

Lesser omentum
(lesser omental sac)

E

Left inferior phrenic artery

Tied branch of left inferior phrenic artery

Belsey's artery

F

Belsey's artery

Left inferior phrenic artery

Mobilization of the entire circumference of the gastroesophageal junction is complete and essential for the performance for either a Mark IV partial fundoplication or a Nissen total fundoplication. Prior to the actual repair, the fat pad at the gastroesophageal junction is resected. This contains a branch of the ascending left gastric artery so that one or more vessels are ligated during the resection of this fatty tissue. Removal of this tissue is essential to allow the gastric serosa to adhere against the esophageal muscle to encourage obliteration and healing of this layer.

Posteriorly, several stitches, usually three, are placed to approximate the crura of the diaphragm. An Allis clamp applied to the tendinous portion of the diaphragm and pulled upward places tension on the origins of the tendinous diaphragm off the vertebral body. This facilitates accurate placement of the medial sutures through tendinous tissue. Laterally, these sutures pass partially through the muscular left crus and exit through the endothoracic fascia to provide substance for the diaphragmatic closure. These sutures are left in place and tied at the end of either the Belsey or the Nissen repair. Up to this point the operative technique is the same for either procedure.

Belsey Mark IV reconstruction. After full mobilization of the cardia and placement of the posterior sutures, the surgeon may choose between a partial fundoplication of the Mark IV type or a total fundoplication. The Belsey Mark IV reconstruction involves the placement of three sutures in each of two rows. The first row of sutures passes through the gastric fundus approximately 2 cm below the junction and obliquely through the longitudinal and circular muscles of the esophagus. The suture is reversed back through the esophagus and the stomach. In this drawing, the first suture is tied laterally near the left vagus nerve. The second mattress suture at the anterior aspect of the fundus and esophagus is being inserted.

When the first row of sutures is complete, the cross-section shows the gastric fundus applied approximately 240 degrees around the circumference of the esophagus. Both vagus nerves are intact posteriorly.

The second row of sutures passes through the tendinous portion of the diaphragm away from the free muscle margin, the fundus of the stomach 2 cm further away from the gastroesophageal junction, and the muscle layers of the esophagus approximately 4 cm above the gastroesophageal junction. All three of these sutures are laid in place before they are tied. A spoon placed on the edge of the diaphragm provides exposure and protection for underlying structures, and avoids the need to make a counter incision in the diaphragm.

At this stage the three sutures of the first row are tied. The left lateral mattress suture in the second row is in place and the middle suture of this second row is being completed.

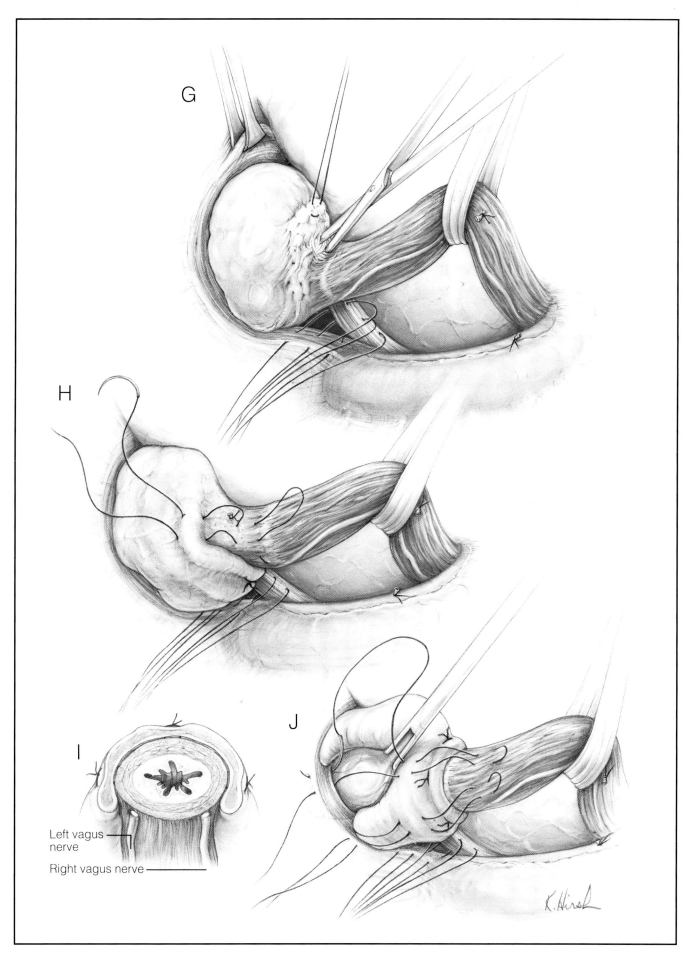

G

H

I

Left vagus nerve

Right vagus nerve

J

K. Hirsh

A cross-section of the reconstruction is shown. Posteriorly the crural sutures provide a buttress against which the intra-abdominal esophagus rests. The first row of mattress sutures between the gastric fundus and esophagus brings approximately 2 cm of distal esophagus within the abdomen. The second row of sutures passing through the diaphragm, gastric fundus, and esophagus completes the 4-cm reduction of an intra-abdominal segment of esophagus. These last sutures are pulled up individually and tied gently so as to not apply too much pressure on the esophageal muscle which might lead to sutures cutting through and causing a recurrence.

The completion of the Belsey Mark IV repair is illustrated with the second row of sutures tied on the thoracic aspect of the diaphragm. After these sutures are placed, the herniated fundus is reduced by hand beneath the diaphragm without tension on the suture. If the esophagus is mobilized adequately up to the aortic arch, this reduction can be accomplished without tension. The pleura is not closed over the mediastinum to enable any fluids which might accumulate to drain from the chest tube.

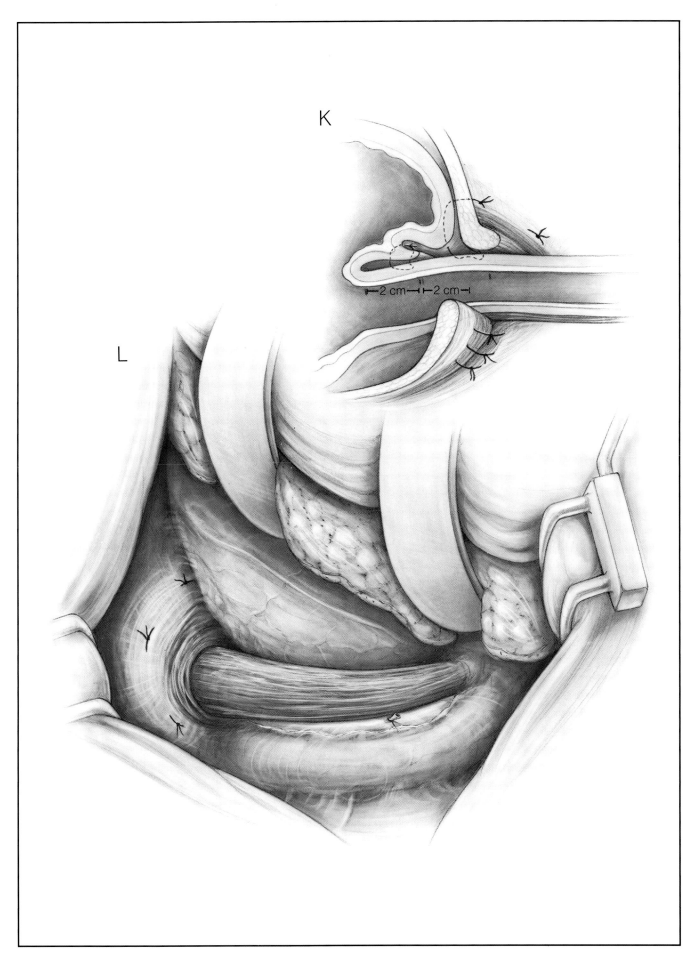

K

L

2 cm 2 cm

# 2 | *Transthoracic Nissen Fundoplication*

**A**  The exposure, mobilization of the cardia, clearing of the fat pad at the cardia, and placement of the posterior diaphragmatic sutures are the same for a transthoracic Nissen fundoplication as it is for the previously illustrated Belsey Mark IV repair. The difference is solely in the way in which the stomach is applied to the intra-abdominal segment of esophagus.

After full mobilization to the aortic arch, short gastric arteries, usually three in number, are ligated and divided to allow the fundus to be brought around the esophagus without tension. In this illustration, a Lockwood clamp is applied to the tip of the fundus near the highest short gastric artery. The esophagus is rotated medial to lateral to allow the sutures to be placed under direct vision and still be on the lesser curvature aspect.

**B**  Sutures are placed between the fundus medially, the esophageal muscles, and the greater curvature tissues laterally to create the fundoplication. It is wise to have a 60 F bougie within the esophagus as the sutures are inserted. The sutures are placed distally first just at the gastroesophageal junction. The fundus is brought around cephalad to the hepatic branch of the vagus nerve. The high gastrohepatic ligament and lesser omentum are left intact. This assures that the wrap will be done on the esophagus and not on the proximal stomach.

As subsequent sutures are placed, the bites in the stomach are moved progressively away from the esophagus as in an inverted pyramid. This rotates more stomach wall within the wrap and ensures that the fundoplication is not too tight at the proximal end. Substantial bites are taken through the longitudinal muscles of the esophagus to anchor the repair securely to the esophagus.

**C**  At the completion of the fundoplication, a 60 F bougie should be in place and passed readily through the cardia. When this is removed, the operator's fingers should easily go down the tunnel adjacent to either vagus nerve.

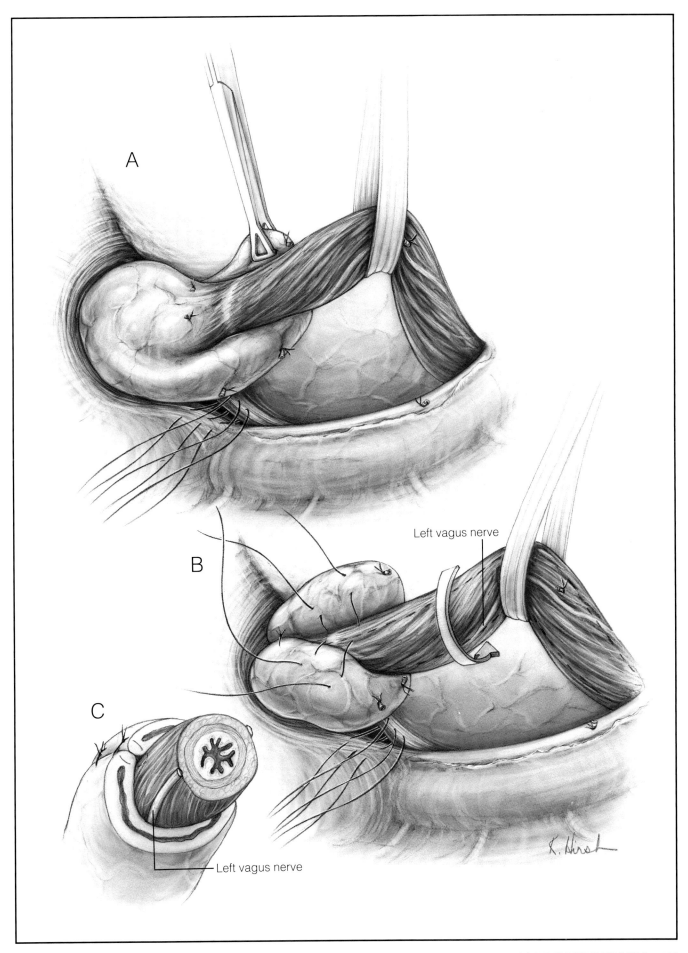

A

B

Left vagus nerve

C

Left vagus nerve

After the fundoplication is in place, the fundus is manually reduced below the diaphragm. With full mobilization of the esophagus up to the aortic arch, this should be achievable without tension. The posterior sutures in the crura are tied to complete the repair.

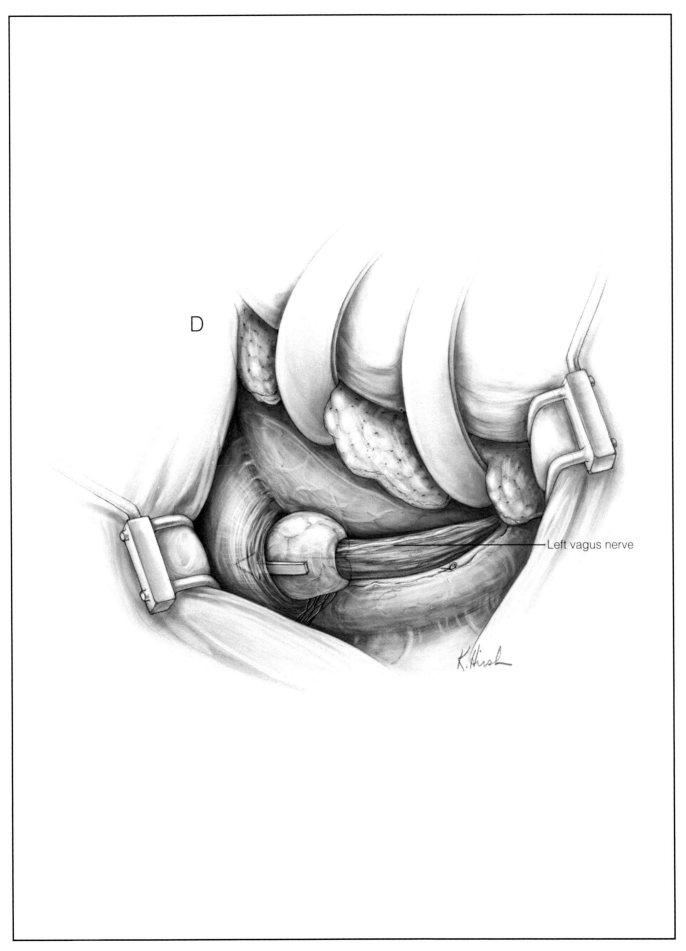

D

Left vagus nerve

K. Hirsh

# 3 | *Transabdominal Antireflux Repairs: Nissen Fundoplication*

**A**    The total fundoplication repair described by Nissen is most commonly done transabdominally. The antireflux repairs introduced by Hill and Guarner are also done transabdominally. An extended right subcostal incision is preferred in most patients.

**B**    After introduction of the upper hand retractor, the gastroesophageal junction is mobilized as shown on pages 4 and 5. A tape, placed around the esophagus, encircles the vagus nerves. For the performance of the total Nissen fundoplication, the highest short gastric arteries between the spleen and stomach are ligated and divided. When this is done, the esophagus should be pulled down and slightly to the left to avoid avulsing any branches of the short gastric vessels from the splenic capsule.

**C**    After the fundus and cardia are mobilized, the crura are approximated with several sutures of 0 silk or a synthetic material. It is essential to identify the intra-abdominal fascia on each pillar of the crura so that the sutures include fascia. If only placed through muscle, there is an increased risk that the ligatures will cut through the tissue. Note that the high gastrohepatic ligament including the hepatic branch of the vagus nerve and any branch of the left gastric artery to the left liver lobe are left intact.

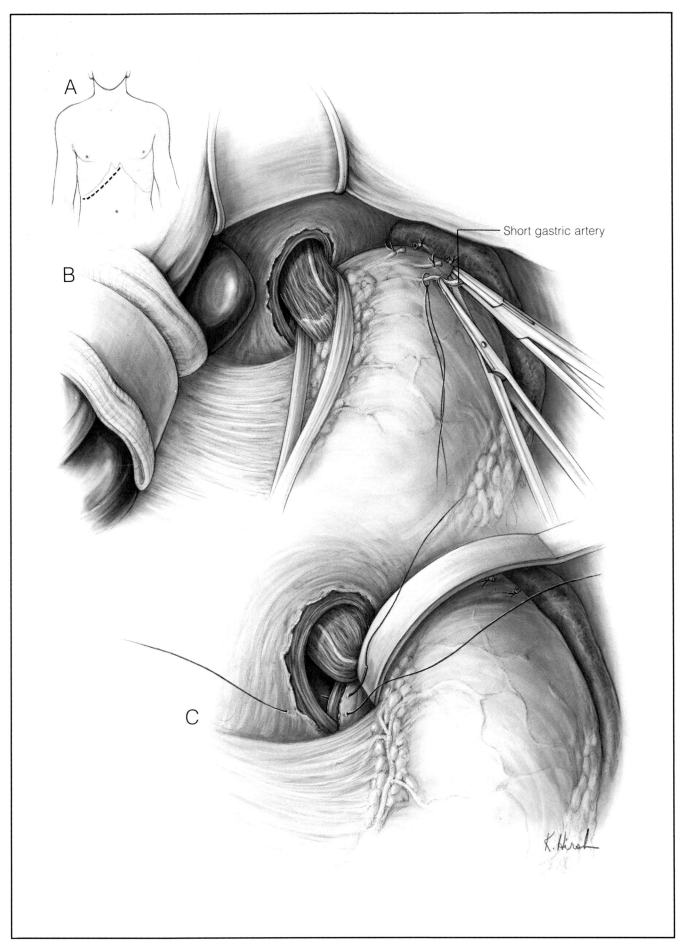

Short gastric artery

The fundus of the stomach is grasped with a Lockwood clamp and pulled behind and around the esophagus. A series of sutures is placed beginning at the gastroesophageal junction and extending cephalad. Each suture is placed through the stomach near the greater curvature on the left side, through the longitudinal muscle of the esophagus, and through the fundus which has been brought posteriorly. As the more proximal sutures are placed they are inserted progressively further away from the esophagus to fold more of the stomach wall behind the esophagus. This avoids making the fundoplication too tight at its upper limit. These sutures are placed with a 60 F bougie within the lumen of the esophagus.

The completed repair is shown. About 3 to 4 cm of distal esophagus are enclosed within the wrap. It is placed above the gastrohepatic ligament which remains intact. The operator's fingers should pass readily along the course of either vagus nerve on either side of the suture line.

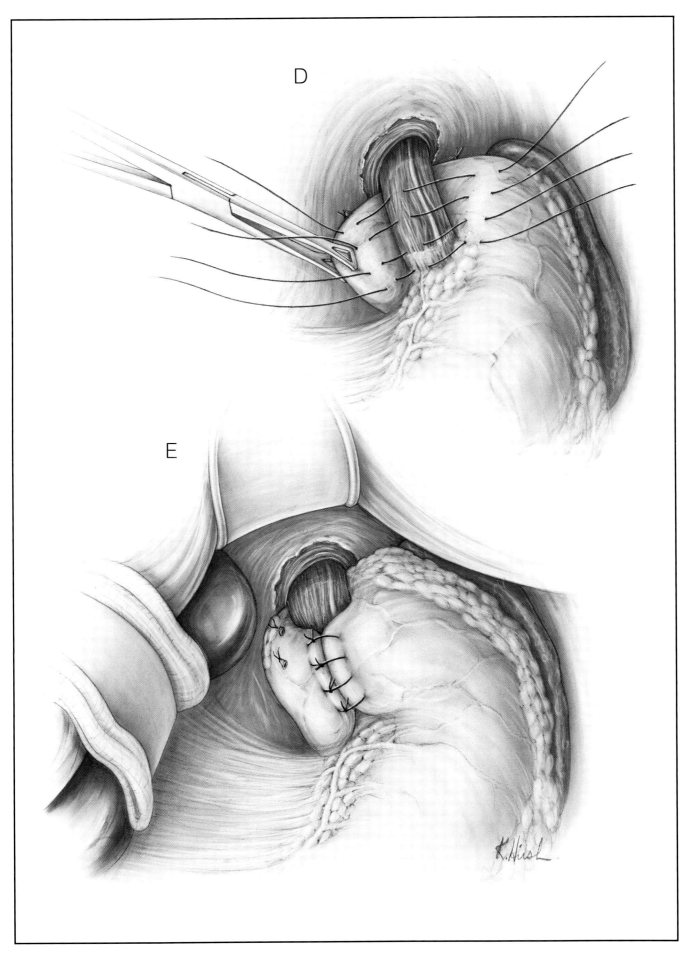

D

E

# 4 | *The Hill Posterior Gastropexy and Calibration of the Cardia*

**A**

This procedure is done transabdominally, and I prefer the extended right subcostal incision in all patients accept for those with a very narrow costal margin.

**B**

After mobilization of the intra-abdominal segment of the esophagus as described previously, the cardia is retracted to the left to identify the arcuate ligament. This ligament passes from the two sides of the vertebral body across the aorta and is the origin of some of the muscle fibers to the diaphragmatic crus. It is best identified by palpating the celiac axis on the aorta that is just caudal to the arcuate ligament. The retroperitoneum and intra-abdominal fascia just above the celiac axis can be incised and the ligament grasped with an Alice clamp.

**C**

An alternate way to identify the arcuate ligament is to pass a finger from within the hiatus behind the origins of the crus and on the surface of the aorta. This draws the crural tissue anteriorly and allows the Alice clamp to be applied to the arcuate ligament.

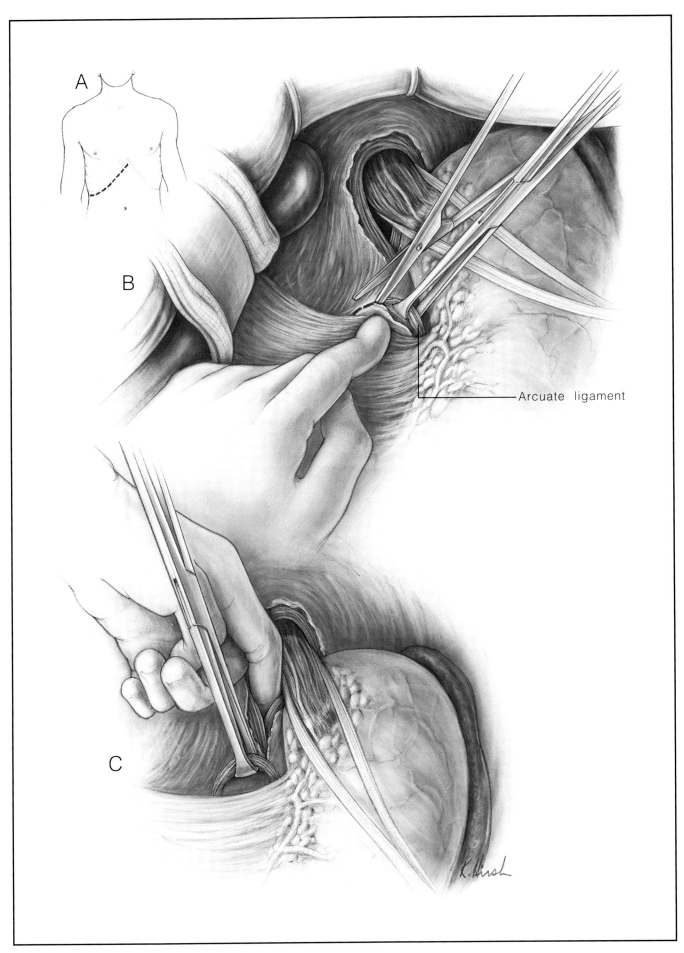

Arcuate ligament

The hiatus is narrowed posteriorly by inserting several stitches, usually three, into the lateral and medial crura being certain to incorporate intra-abdominal fascia. The Hill posterior gastropexy is started by placing a 2-0 silk or synthetic suture with swedged on needle through the bundle of tissue on the right posterior aspect of the gastroesophageal junction that represents the superior extent of the gastrohepatic ligament. A substantial amount of tissue is obtained. The needle passes through the left edge of the arcuate ligament. This is the principle gastrepexy suture.

The fibrofatty tissue around the gastroesophageal junction both anteriorly and posteriorly is grasped. Calibration of the cardia is performed by placing sutures through the tissue on the left anterior and right posterior aspects of the cardia and then passing the suture through the arcuate ligament. The first or lower suture is passed through the right inferior margin of the arcuate ligament.

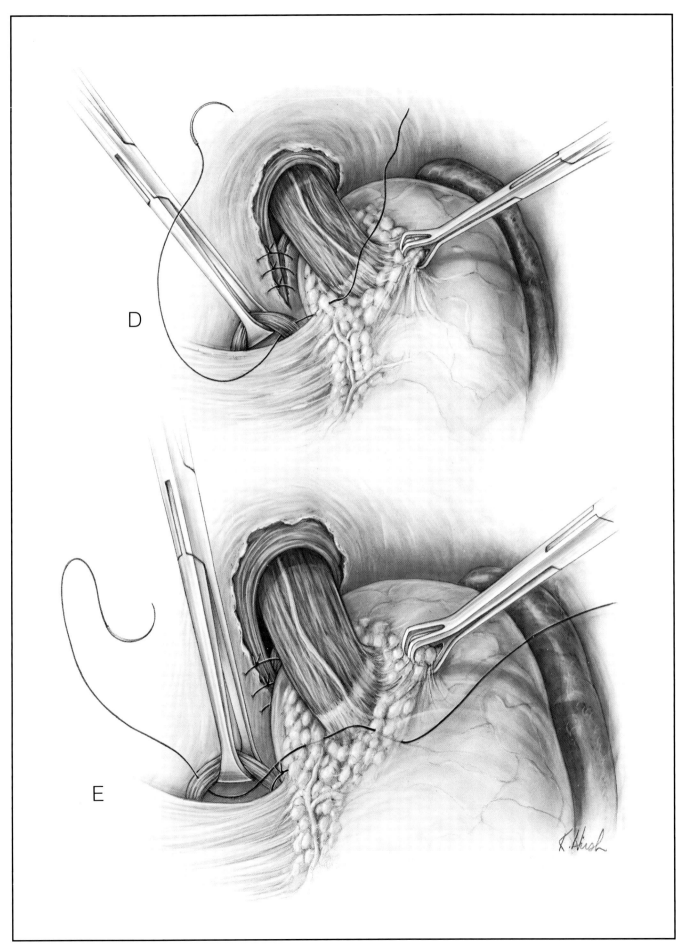

D

E

**F** Two or three additional sutures are passed through the pillars of fibrofatty tissues surrounding the cardia and through the arcuate ligament in a step-wise fashion. A manometric assembly is passed by the anesthesiologist through the nose and down the esophagus into the stomach. As each of these sutures is tied, a recording of pressures in the reconstruction is made. Intraoperative findings are that the closure of the hiatus posteriorly does not affect intraluminal pressure at the cardia. However, the calibration sutures should raise intraluminal pressure to the level of approximately 50 mmHg. If pressures in excess of at least 30 mmHg are not obtained, reflux will not be controlled. If pressure exceeds 60 mmHg, the patient may have postoperative dysphagia.

**G** After the several calibrations sutures are tied, final pressures are recorded once again. If 30 to 50 mmHg are recorded, the Hill posterior gastropexy and calibration of the cardia is complete. It represents a partial anterior fundoplication around the intra-abdominal segment of esophagus.

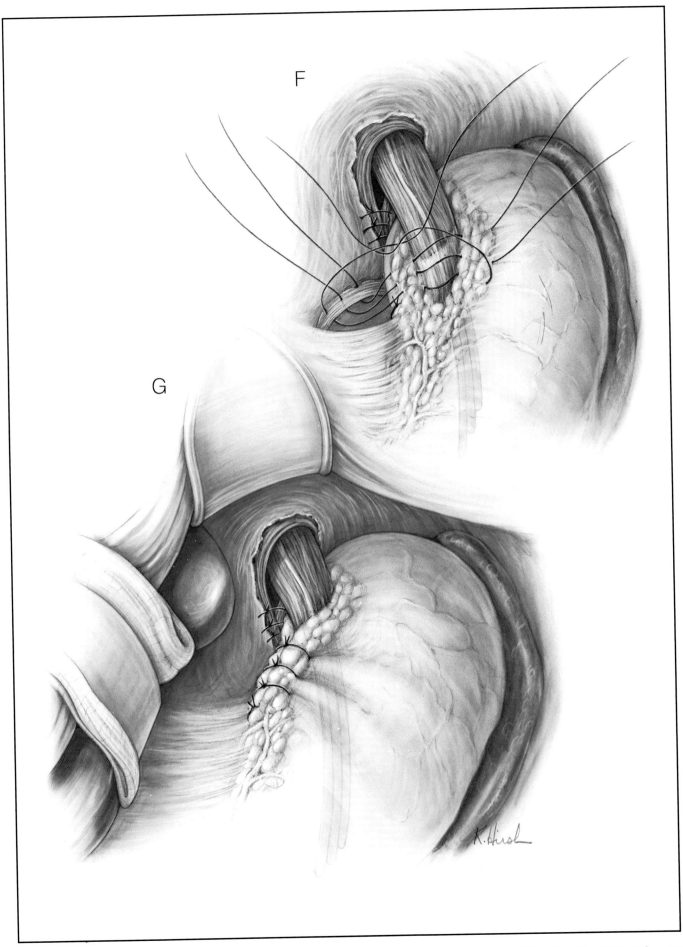

# 5 | *The Guarner Partial Fundoplication*

**A**

The Guarner partial fundoplication is performed through an abdominal incision.

**B**

After mobilization of the intra-abdominal esophagus, sutures are placed to narrow the hiatus posteriorly.

**C**

After division of several short gastric vessels, the fundus is brought behind the esophagus. Two rows of sutures are placed between the fundus on the right and the anterior surfaces of the stomach and on the left between the gastric serosa and the esophageal muscle. This intra-abdominal segment of esophagus prevents overdistension of the distal esophagus during periods of gastric distension. Results achieved with this repair are comparable to those achieved with the previously described repairs. Because this is not a full fundoplication, the incidence of postoperative dysphagia is less than with a Nissen total wrap.

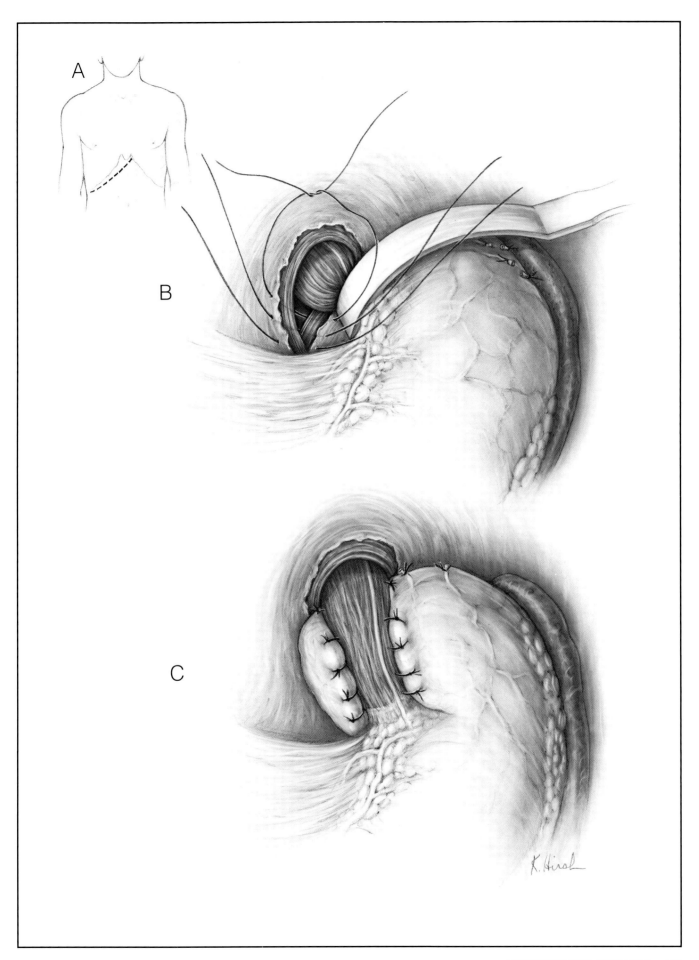

# CHAPTER VI

# *Strictures*

Reflux-induced acid peptic strictures of the distal esophagus occur at the squamocolumnar junction and represent an advanced stage of reflux esophagitis. In patients in whom the strictures are difficult to dilate or that have recurred after previous antireflux surgery, resection of the distal esophagus may be necessary. Reconstruction after such a resection may be accomplished with colon or jejunal interposition as described in Chapter III. Other procedures short of resection may be employed to treat strictures when an antireflux repair cannot be successfully accomplished because of shortening and scarring of the esophagus. In our practice, it is rare for these procedures to be necessary as a first operation. Intensive medical therapy and dilatation of the stricture usually permits successful performance of an antireflux repair.

# 1 | The Collis Gastroplasty and Antireflux Repair

This procedure is employed when the surgeon feels that an antireflux repair will be under too much tension due to esophageal shortening. The concept is to lengthen the swallowing tube by cutting a cylinder of stomach along the lesser curvature as an extension of the esophagus.

*A*  The operation is usually done through a left thoracotomy using the same approach for mobilization of the esophagus and cardia as described for the transthoracic antireflux repairs.

*B*  A bougie as large as may be accommodated by the stricture is passed by mouth through the esophagus into the stomach.

*C*  Short gastric vessels are divided similar to the method for a thoracic Nissen fundoplication. A tube of lesser curvature of 5 cm in length is prepared. The fundus and greater curvature are pulled up tautly and a stapler or clamps are applied exactly parallel to the axis of the esophagus with the bougie in place.

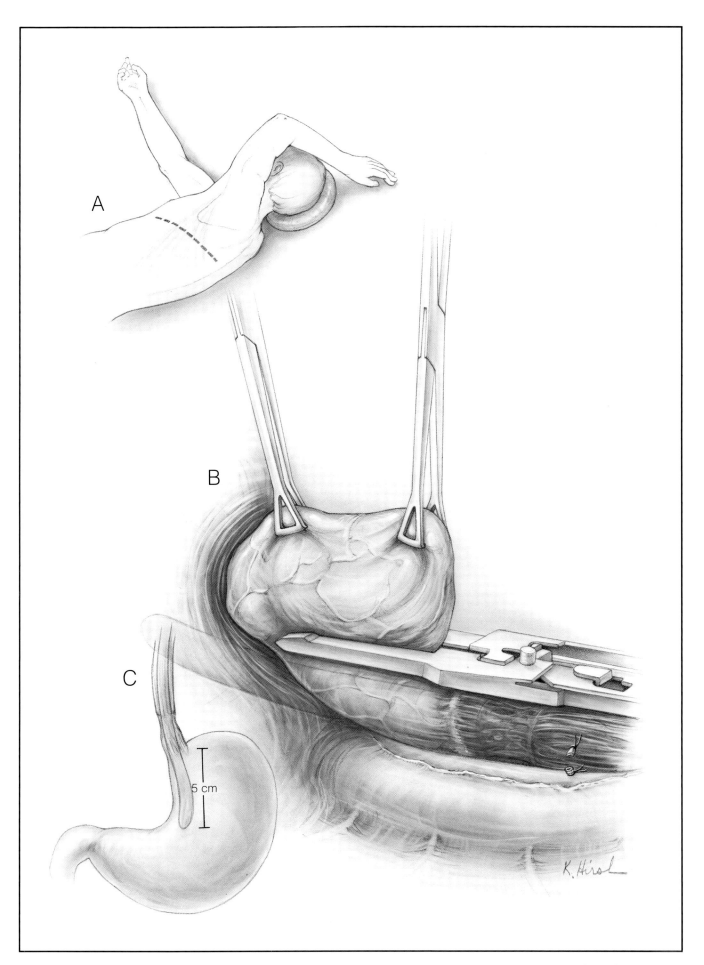

After the fundus is divided from the lesser curvature with the stapler or clamps, an elongation of the swallowing tube is achieved. Care is taken that the tube is not narrowed at this distal end causing dysphagia, or does not flare like an inverted funnel causing increased likelihood of reflux.

The staple or hemostatic suture line is turned in with running seromuscular sutures.

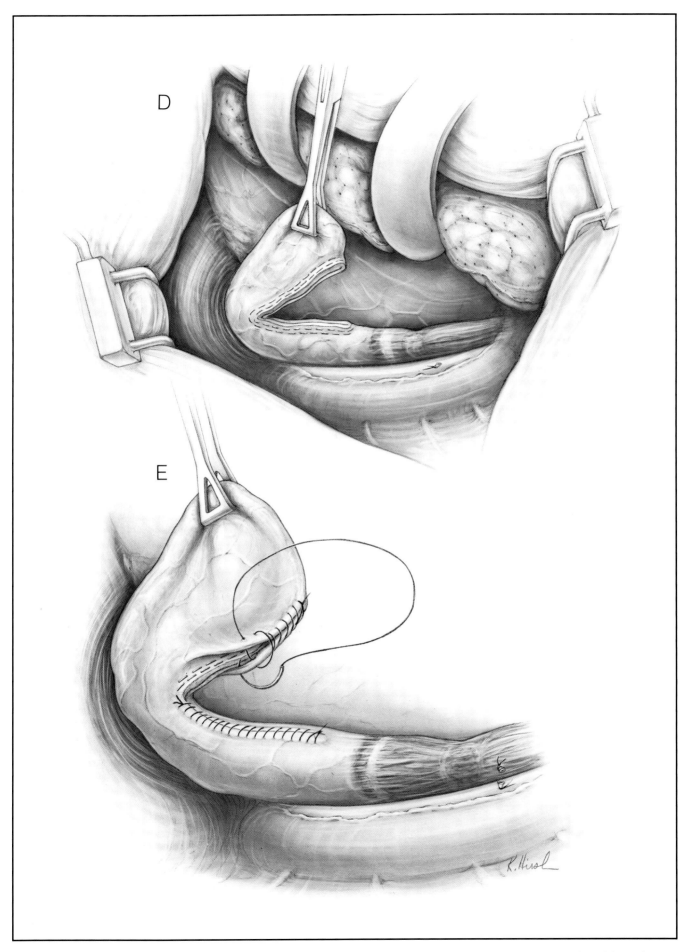

D

E

Steps in the creation of a total fundo-plication around the gastric tube are illustrated.

The antireflux repair is constructed using the new fundus and elongated swallowing tube. Either a circumfer-ential Nissen fundoplication or par-tial Mark IV type repair may be em-ployed. Sutures are again placed in the diaphragmatic hiatus posteriorly. The fundus may be wrapped around the tube and sutured to itself as a to-tal fundoplication. Some surgeons prefer to do this with the gastroplasty tube stapled but uncut and included in the wrap.

Alternatively, a partial fundoplica-tion of the Mark IV type may be per-formed. At this stage, the first row of three mattress sutures have been placed. The fundus is rotated slightly so the gastric tube suture line and fundus lines do not touch each other. The second row of sutures between the diaphragm, fundus, and gastric tube is being inserted.

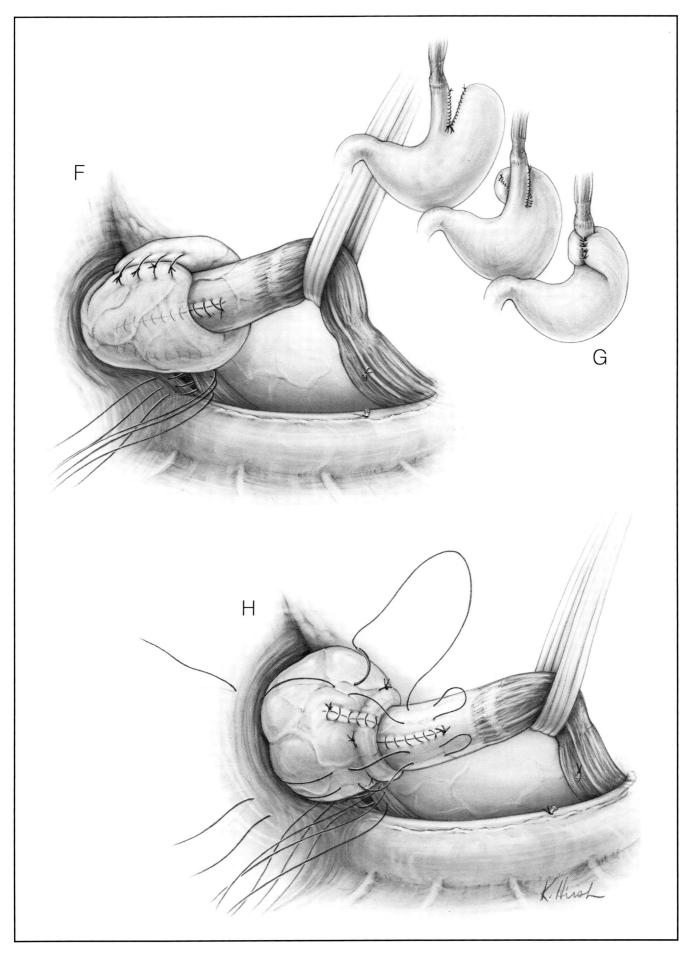

# 2 | *Thal Patch and Antireflux Repair*

This procedure, described by Thal, involves cutting across the stricture and applying a skin graft. An antireflux repair is done over the grafted esophagus.

**A**    This operation is performed through a left sixth interspace thoracotomy.

**B**    After full mobilization of the esophagus and cardia, the stricture region is incised full thickness into the lumen and allowed to gape open.

**C**    A partial-thickness skin graft is laid over the defect with the epithelial side facing the lumen. This is sutured in place circumferentially. A bougie is inserted to maintain the lumen of the esophagus while the patch is applied.

**D**    With the bougie still in place, a full fundoplication is performed. Posterior crural sutures are inserted. This repair is replaced beneath the diaphragm if possible. Alternately, it can be left in the chest and treated as an intrathoracic Nissen fundoplication (see pages 150 to 153).

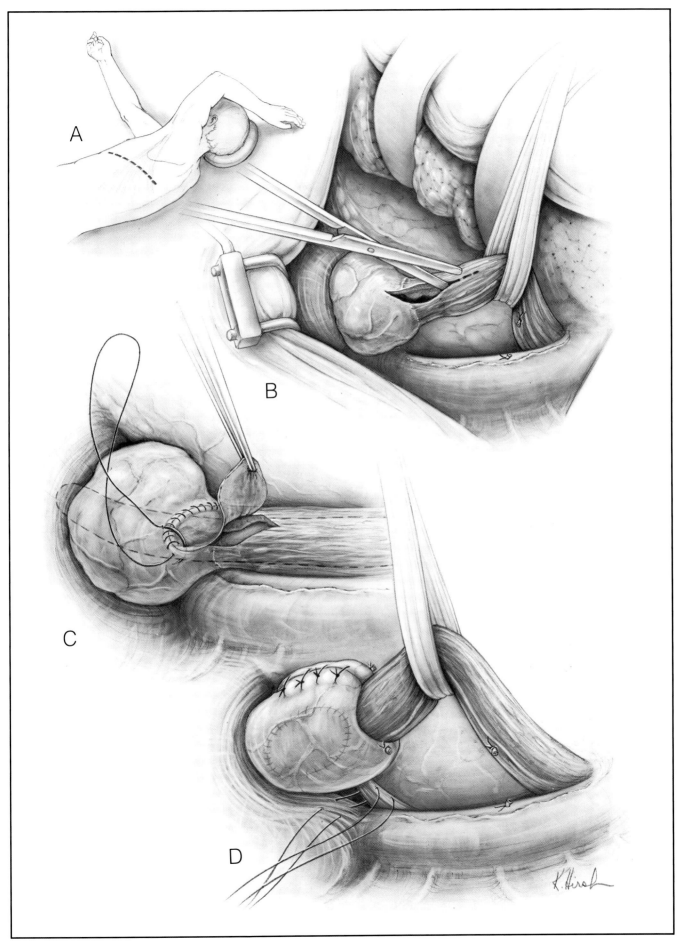

# 3 | *Intrathoracic Total Fundoplication*

Occasionally a full Nissen fundoplication is performed but cannot be reduced into the abdomen because of esophageal shortening. This may also be the case when a Thal fundic patch is applied. If the fundoplication is circumferential, it may be left within the chest if certain steps are taken.

The procedure is done through a left thoracotomy.

After the fundoplication is complete, and it is apparent that it does not readily reduce into the abdomen, a cuff of diaphragm is excised around the free margin of the hiatus. This is done to enlarge the hiatus and prevent an hourglass deformity on the fundus and body of the stomach. The diaphragm may either be enlarged with radial cuts or a portion excised. The use of the spoon retractor protects the underlying organs from injury by cautery.

The hiatus should be enlarged sufficiently for the operator's hand to pass through. This prevents any risk of obstruction to the intrathoracic gastric pouch.

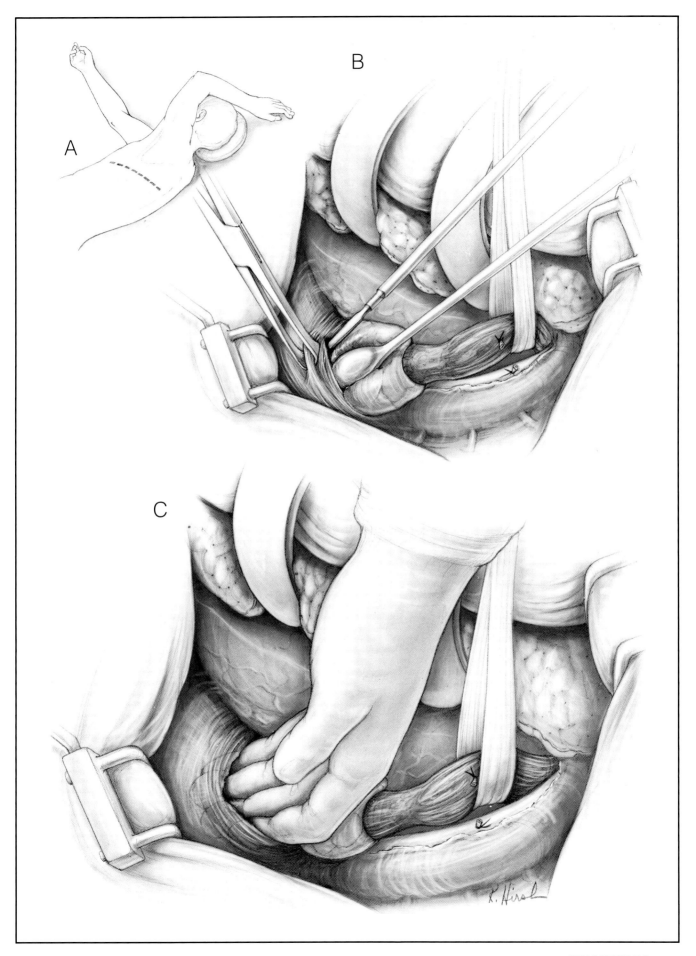

The intrathoracic total fundoplication is securely anchored to the margins of the hiatus with numerous interrupted sutures through the seromuscular layer of the stomach and the margins of the hiatus. This is done to prevent further gastric herniation into the chest or herniation of small intestine along side the stomach. This leaves an iatrogenic hiatus hernia in the chest which tends to enlarge over time unless the stomach is securely fixed. Sutures are also placed between the tip of the gastric wrap and esophagus to prevent the esophagus from evaginating from the fundoplication into the negative intrathoracic pressure environment.

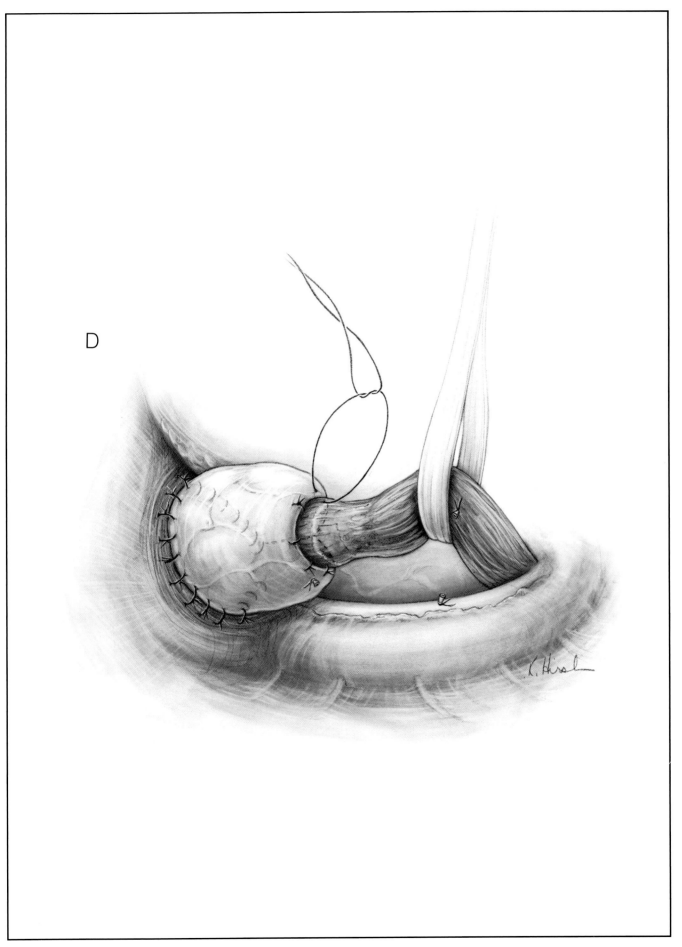

D

# *Motor Disorders*

Motor disorders are characterized by muscular dysfunction so that a myotomy is a portion of the treatment for these diseases.

# 1 | *Achalasia*

**A**

Treatment for achalasia includes a long esophagomyotomy and partial fundoplication to prevent reflux. The operation is usually done through a left thoracotomy, but can be approached transabdominally.

**B**

Through the left thoracotomy, the esophagus and cardia are mobilized as for an antireflux repair. The myotomy is started on the body of the esophagus. The muscle layers are lifted up with forceps, and scissors are used to begin the myotomy. The pinching action of the scissors forces the mucosa away as it is approached, making this technique safer than using a scalpel. As illustrated, there is normally a branch of the vagus nerve crossing from medial to lateral in a cranial to caudal direction. This is mobilized off the muscle and retracted using a suture. Care is taken not to touch vagus nerve branches with metallic instruments.

**C**

The myotomy is extended proximally to the aortic arch or to the level where the thickened muscle becomes more normal. Distally the myotomy is continued across the gastroesophageal junction and 1 to 2 cm onto the stomach to be certain that all circular fibers are divided. When this is completed, an antireflux repair is performed. One or two sutures are used to narrow the hiatus posteriorly but this must not be snug.

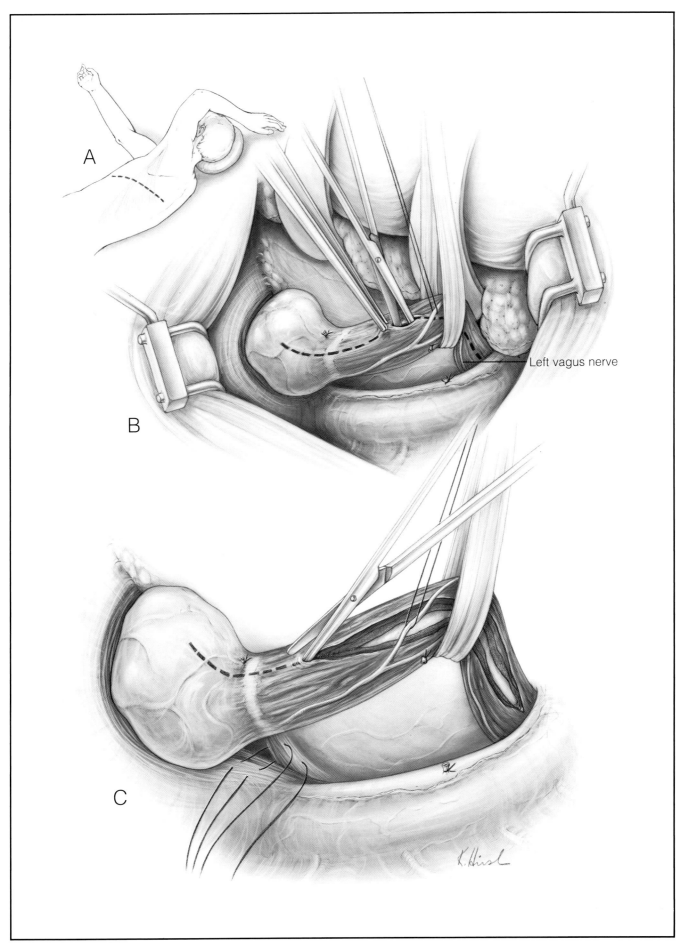

Left vagus nerve

After the myotomy is complete, the edges of the muscle are dissected back from the mucosa using blunt dissection. Approximately one-half of the circumference of the mucosal tube should be exposed. This prevents the muscle edges being pulled together by fibrosis during the healing process.

 A modified Mark IV antireflux repair is performed to prevent postoperative reflux through the widened cardia. The middle suture in the standard repair is eliminated as this would be located in the region of the myotomy. The first row of two sutures adjacent to each vagus nerve is tied. Their placement is shown in Figure D. The second row of sutures is placed through the tendinous portion of the diaphragm, gastric fundus, and esophageal muscle approximately 5 cm above the gastroesophageal junction. If the esophagus is very dilated and redundant, a longer length of intra-abdominal esophagus can be created by placing the sutures higher leading to some straightening out of a sigmoid shaped esophagus.

 The completed myotomy and antireflux repair is illustrated. Placing the two sutures through the diaphragm as far around the circumference of the hiatus as possible encourages gaping of the mucosal tube within the fundoplication. Since the esophagus does not contract longitudinally with achalasia, recurrence of reflux or hiatal hernia after this approach is nearly nonexistent.

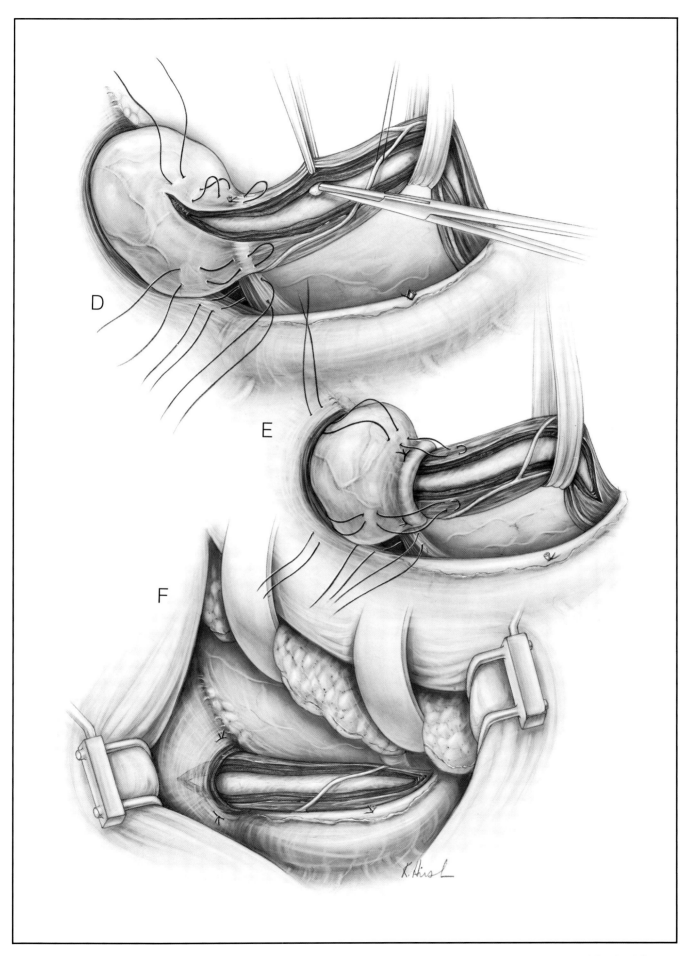

# 2 | *Diffuse Esophageal Spasm*

In patients with diffuse esophageal spasm of an idiopathic nature, myotomy may be helpful if the principle complaint is dysphagia. Myotomy is rarely successful in eliminating pain from diffuse esophageal spasm.

In this disorder the circular muscle is extremely thickened (as much as 2 cm in thickness). Myotomy should extend the full length of the thickened muscle and must cross the cardia to eliminate any obstruction at the lower end of the myotomy. The muscle edges are dissected well back to expose a considerable portion of the circumference of the mucosal tube. This is particularly important in diffuse esophageal spasm as high pressure muscle contractions are capable of bursting the mucosal tube postoperatively if the muscle is able to grip much of the circumference of the mucosa. An antireflux repair of the modified Mark IV type similar to that for achalasia completes the procedure.

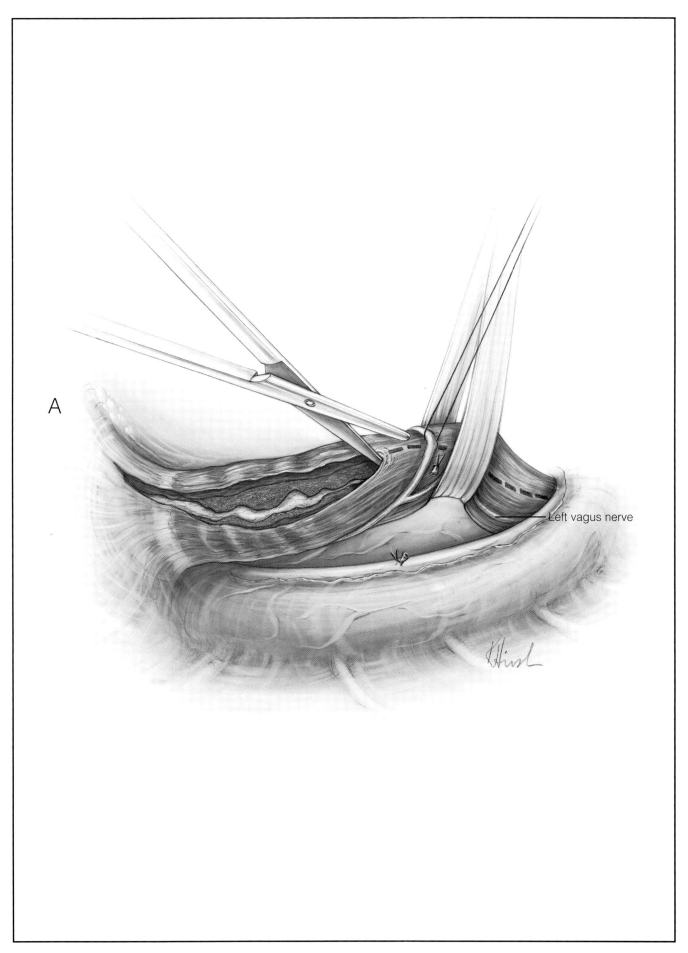

A

Left vagus nerve

# 3 | *Zenker's Diverticulum*

A protrusion of mucosa cephalad to the cricopharyngeal sphincter is the most common diverticulum of the pharynx and esophagus.

The approach is through a cervical incision by extending to one side or the other of the midline. Right handed surgeons may prefer to approach this from the left side, although the thoracic duct is more exposed to injury by this approach. The incision is completed as shown on pages 12 to 15.

After the esophagus is exposed and the prevertebral fascia is dissected, the diverticulum is evident in the posterior mediastinum. Exposure is improved by tension on the stay suture placed through the strap muscle and thyroid gland. No retractors are placed medially to avoid injury to the recurrent laryngeal nerves.

The tip of the diverticulum is grasped with a noncrushing Lockwood clamp or held with a stay suture. The muscle and fibrous tissue on the diverticulum are dissected back so that the mucosal pouch of the diverticulum is fully exposed to its neck.

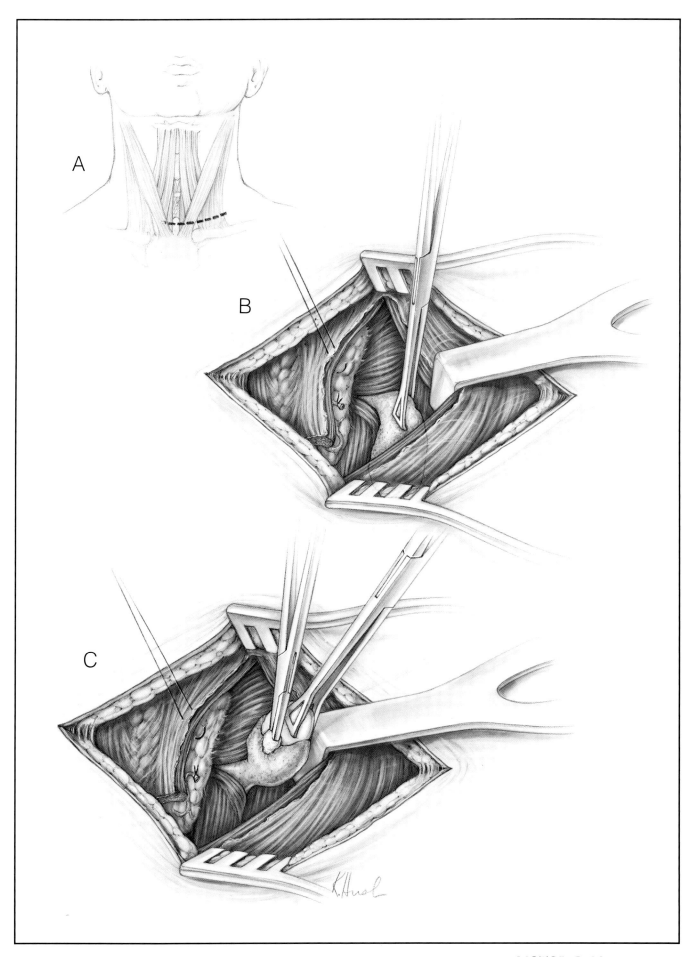

The myotomy is started on the esophagus posterolaterally below the region of the cricopharyngeal sphincter. The myotomy is carried distally to the thoracic inlet. The tracheoesophageal groove is avoided to prevent injury to the recurrent laryngeal nerve. As illustrated by the dotted line, the myotomy is carried up to the neck of the diverticulum and slightly onto the inferior constrictor of the hypopharynx.

When the myotomy is complete, the mucosal cylinder from the pharynx down should balloon freely through the cut muscle edges. A biopsy may be taken from the sphincter muscle. A tube is passed by the anesthesiologist into the upper esophagus and insufflated with air to demonstrate that there are no residual fibers, obstruction, or pinhole leaks.

The pouch is suspended upside down to the prevertebral fascia with one or more sutures. In the case illustrated, the pouch is large and is being effaced against the prevertebral fascia by five mattress sutures placed in horseshoe fashion. When these are tied, the tube is again passed back and forth through the pharynx into the esophagus to demonstrate that there is no obstruction. If the procedure is done under local anesthesia, the patient is asked to drink liquids at this point to demonstrate free passage.

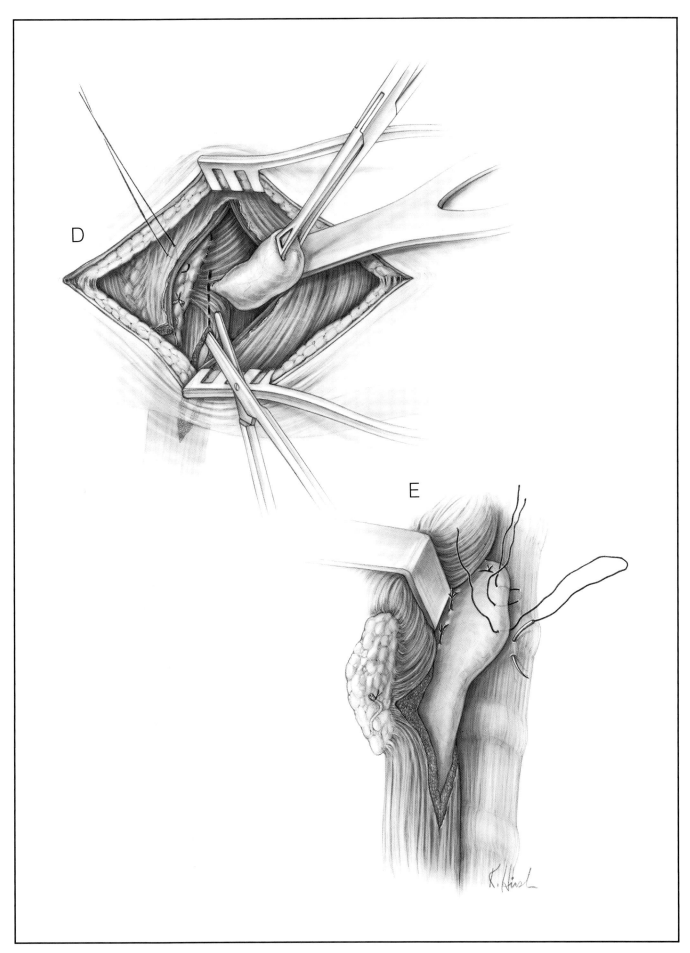

D

E

# 4 | *Epiphrenic Diverticulum*

In nearly all cases of epiphrenic diverticulum there is a demonstrable motor disorder. The diverticulum is viewed as secondary to dysfunction of the distal esophageal muscle.

**A** Even though the diverticulum usually presents into the right chest, the operation is performed through a left thoracotomy to provide optimal exposure to the distal esophagus as it enters the hiatus.

**B** The esophagus is fully mobilized starting at the level of the inferior pulmonary vein. The right side pleura is bluntly dissected off the esophagus until the neck of the diverticulum is identified.

The esophagus just at the region of the hiatus is similarly mobilized and dissected staying very close to the phrenoesophageal membrane. Tapes are passed around the esophagus cephalad and caudal to the diverticulum to be elevated up out of the mediastinum. With blunt dissection, the right pleura is pushed off the diverticulum which is completed delivered into the left chest. This is facilitated by entering the peritoneum at the esophageal hiatus so that a portion of the stomach can be drawn up to increase the freedom of the esophageal mobilization.

**C** As shown, the diverticulum usually protrudes from the right posterior aspect of the esophagus into the right chest behind the right vagus nerve.

**D** **E** The diverticulum is delivered into the left chest and rotated so that its entire base can be visualized. This rotates the esophagus approximately 180 degrees and brings the right vagus nerve into the preaortic location. The splayed out muscular and fibrous tissue over the diverticulum is dissected back to the neck of the diverticulum leaving just the mucosal pouch intact. This is continued until the free edges of the muscular defect are clearly identified.

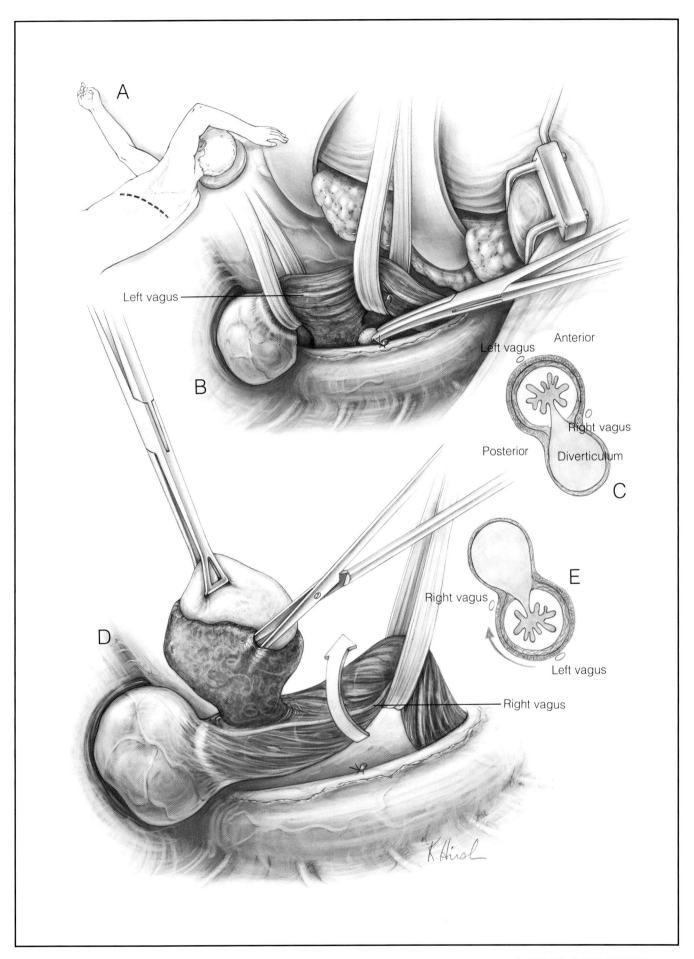

A

Left vagus

B

Anterior

Left vagus

Right vagus

Posterior

Diverticulum

C

E

Right vagus

Left vagus

Right vagus

D

K. Hirsh

**F** Once the neck of the diverticulum is identified circumferentially in the submucosal plane, preparations are made to resect a large diverticulum. A 60 F bougie is placed through the esophagus into the stomach to avoid narrowing of the lumen during the resection. Stay sutures are placed at the upper and lower limits of the anticipated mucosal incision. The resection is done leaving enough cuff of mucosa free from the lumen distended by the dilator so that a closure can be done without narrowing the mucosal cylinder.

**G** A schematic demonstration of the closure with the sutures tied on the inside of the lumen using a single layer full-thickness suture technique.

**H** The sutures are started at the upper and lower ends of the incision being certain to include a good bit of mucosa in each. After several sutures are placed, the final closure sutures are tied on the outside of the esophagus.

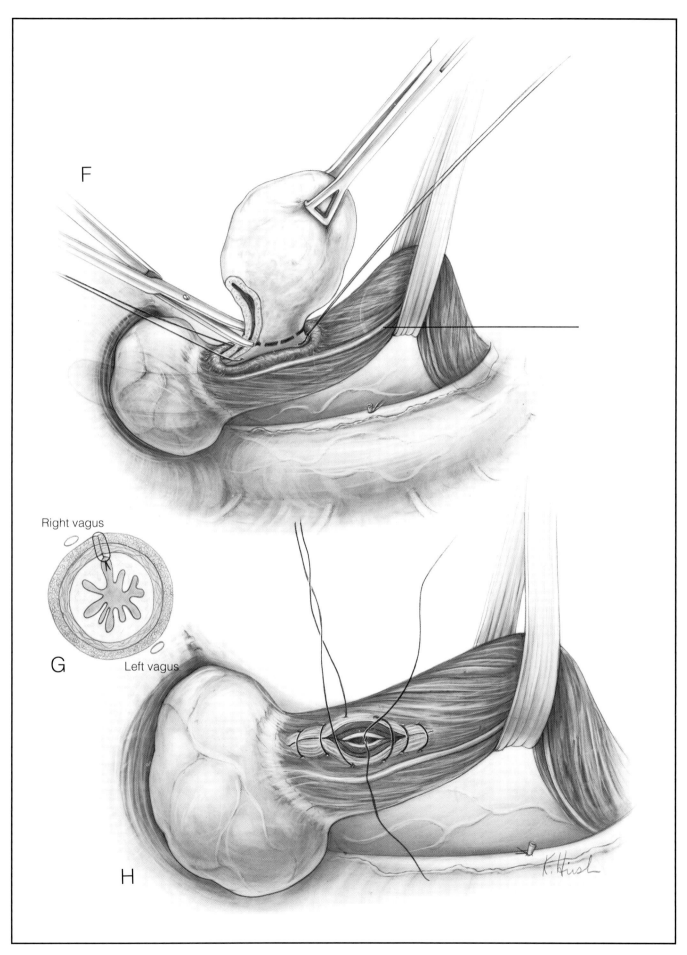

F

Right vagus

G

Left vagus

H

**I** After the base of the diverticulum is closed, the esophagus is allowed to rotate back to its normal location placing the suture line to the right and away from and out of view of the surgeon.

**J** Since the diverticulum is almost always associated with a motor disorder, a myotomy is done in the standard fashion on the left anterolateral aspect of the esophagus 180 degrees away from the suture line. The myotomy must be carried down and on to the stomach for a centimeter or so to be sure that all distal obstruction below the suture line is eliminated. The myotomy is carried superiorly to the level of the top of the diverticulum or higher if the muscle is thickened or preoperative manometry shows a more proximal motor disorder.

**K** Schematically, a cross-section illustrates the closure of the diverticulum toward the right and the myotomy on the left anterior surface. The myotomy extending onto the stomach will cause reflux so a partial fundoplication of stomach is done as for achalasia.

**L** The first row of two sutures on either side of the myotomy and near the vagus nerves have been inserted. This figure illustrates the placement of the sutures in the second row through the diaphragm, gastric fundus, and esophageal wall. When these are tied, the reconstruction is placed below the diaphragm. The crural sutures are tied to complete the operation.

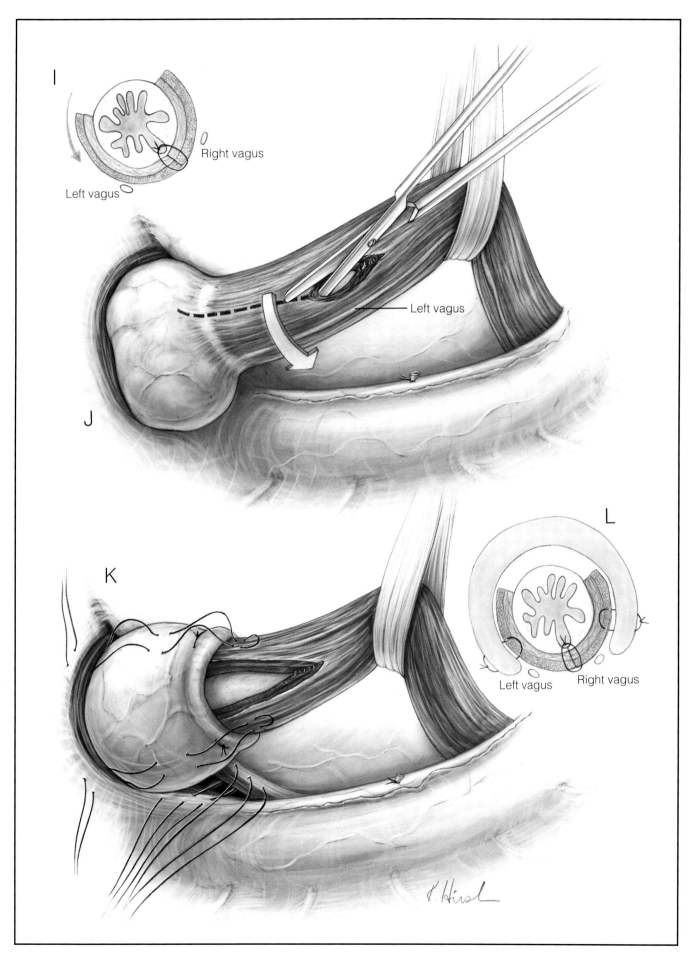

I

Left vagus

Right vagus

J

Left vagus

K

L

Left vagus

Right vagus

# 5 | *Leiomyoma*

Leiomyoma is the most common nonmalignant tumor of the esophagus. It frequently presents with symptoms of chest pain or dysphagia and is often encountered during the evaluation of the patient for a possible motor disorder. Occasionally a motor disorder is associated with a leiomyoma, and its management is therefore included in this section.

**A** The operative approach is dictated by the level of the tumor determined endoscopically. If it is in the distal esophagus, a left thoracotomy is preferred. A middle or upper third leiomyoma is approached through a right thoracotomy.

**B** The leiomyoma almost always lies within the circular muscle of the esophagus and presents as a bolus under the mucosa. A suspected leiomyoma should not be biopsied endoscopically before surgery, but the mucosa is inspected to be certain that it is intact.

**C** An incision is made through the overlying longitudinal and circular muscle until the surface of the tumor is encountered. These tumors are almost always encapsulated and can be freed away from the underlying submucosa and muscle. If the tumor appears to be invasive, a sarcoma must be suspected.

**D** The tumor is elevated through the gap in the muscle and the mucosa is gently dissected away. Should the mucosa be entered, it would be closed as illustrated previously for the resection of a diverticulum; however, this is a rare event in the resection of a leiomyoma.

**E** If the leiomyoma is extensive, the muscle may be closed with interrupted or running sutures. If the defect is small, closure is not necessary. Unless a concomitant motor disorder has been diagnosed by preoperative manometry, there is no need to extend the myotomy proximally or distally from the region of the tumor.

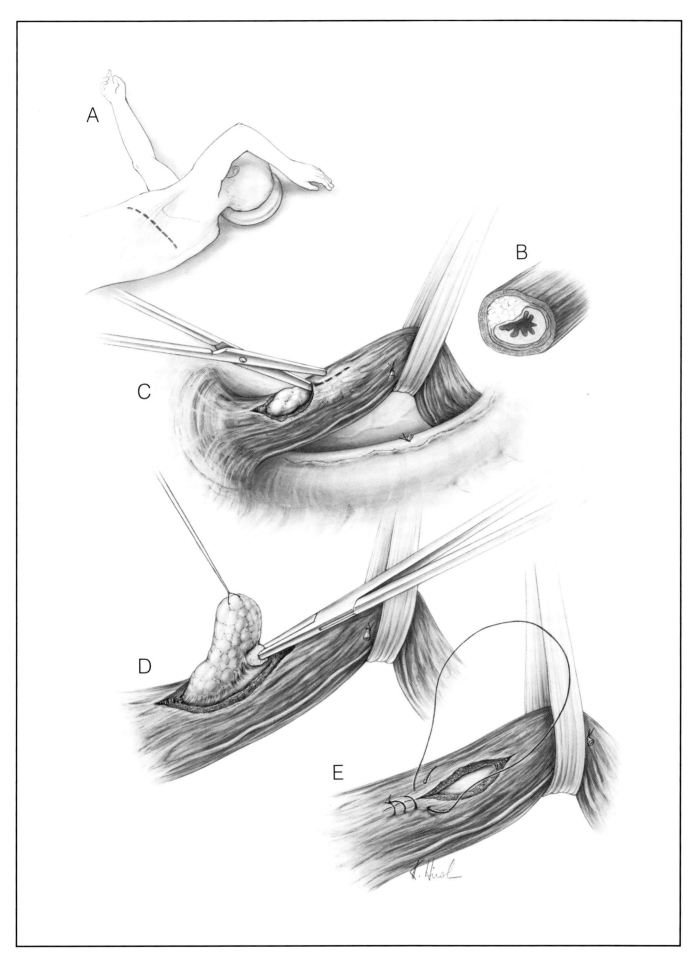

# *Esophageal Rupture*

There are a number of causes for esophageal rupture including spontaneous, instrumental perforation, penetrating trauma, or an underlying disease process such as Barrett's ulcer or neoplasia. In the latter instances, an esophageal resection and reconstruction may be necessary. For perforation of an esophagus previously normal before the rupture, options include primary repair, esophageal exclusion, and rarely resection if the injury is extensive.

# 1 | *Primary Repair with Pleural Patch*

**A** Spontaneous rupture of the esophagus most commonly occurs in the distal third and is approached through a thoracotomy on the side in which the rupture has presented. In this case a left thoracotomy is illustrated.

**B** The rupture is seen as a rent in the overlying pleura with bruised and edematous esophageal muscle overlying the tear.

**C** The esophagus is mobilized from the mediastinum to improve exposure. The muscle is always in spasm, and the muscular defect is always less extensive than the mucosal tear underneath. For this reason the tear in the muscle should be extended by incision proximally and distally until the full extent of the mucosal tear can be seen and the edges identified.

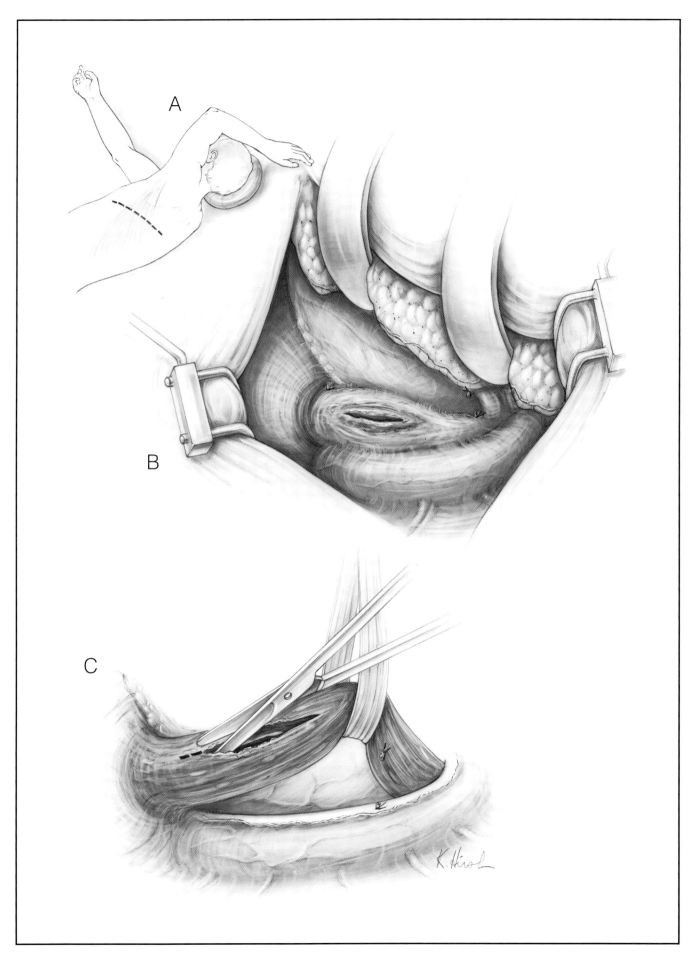

If the perforation is diagnosed promptly and operation undertaken within 12 to 24 hours, the quality of the esophageal mucosa and muscle is such that a primary repair can be undertaken. Full-thickness single layer interrupted sutures are placed with the knots tied on the inside of the esophagus. Care must be taken with each bite to include a generous amount of esophageal mucosa as the submucosa is the only layer having sufficient strength to hold sutures.

If there is any doubt about the quality of the tissues, and this is usually the case, the closure may be reinforced with a patch. This might be done with adjacent diaphragm or stomach if the esophagus is ruptured in the region of the cardia and an antireflux repair is required. At other levels, a pleural patch works effectively. A long patch is prepared by elevating pleura from the chest wall near the incision back to the base of the aorta.

The patch is placed circumferentially around the esophagus to cover the suture line and held gently in place with tacking sutures. It is not clear as to whether the pleural patch requires attachment at its base and remains vascularized, but is probably wise to do so. The chest is closed with drainage, and the lung must be fully expanded with all foreign material irrigated from the pleura.

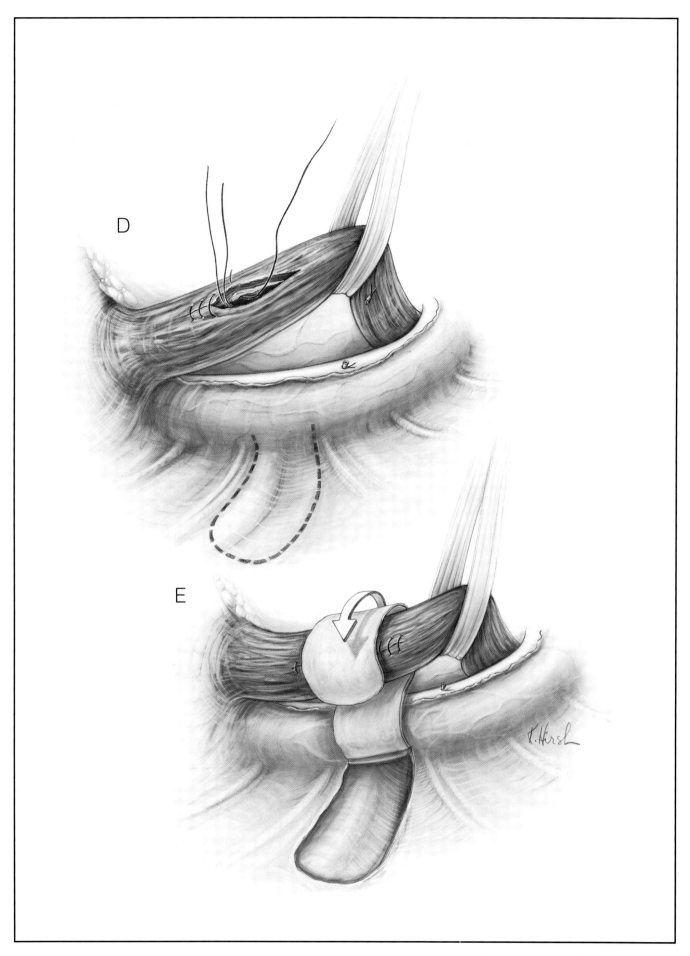

D

E

# 2 | *Esophageal Diversion*

When the esophageal rupture is not diagnosed promptly and infection is well established, it is unlikely that a primary repair will be successful. Unless underlying neoplasia or ulceration dictates the necessity for a resection, esophagectomy is avoided as being unduly hazardous in the face of extensive sepsis. Under these circumstances, esophageal diversion is performed dividing the organ in the neck with an end-esophagostomy.

The diagram illustrates division of the esophagus at the level of the sternal manubrium bringing the proximal end out to the skin where it is matured. The distal esophagus in the neck is closed and attached to the back of the esophageal stoma so that it can be easily found at the time of reconstruction. Distal to this closure line, a catheter is inserted through a pursestring suture in the side of the esophagus and brought out through a stab wound on the opposite side of the neck. This provides drainage of the esophagus, and prevents mucous accumulation keeping the fistula open.

A laparotomy is performed and the cardia is closed. Interrupted interlocking mattress sutures are more secure than a circular ligature which leads to muscle necrosis and re-establishment of the channel. A gastrostomy is inserted using the 26 Foley catheter with 30 cc balloon. A double pursestring suture secures the catheter which is pulled up to the abdominal wall. Interrupted stitches between the gastric serosa and peritoneum in four quadrants secure the opening to the peritoneum. The catheter is further sutured at the skin level.

For additional security and nutritional purposes, a feeding jejunostomy may be inserted in the first jejunal loop through a double pursestring suture. This is in turn anchored to the peritoneum with several interrupted sutures, and the tube is again fixed at the skin level.

If the esophageal rupture is demonstrated to close by inserting a small amount of contrast material through the drainage tube in the neck 4 to 6 weeks later, the esophagostomy may be closed by an end-to-end anastomosis and the sutures at the cardia removed. Occasionally it may be necessary to perform an anastomosis between the distal esophagus and the stomach if the lumen is scarred by a ligature or sutures.

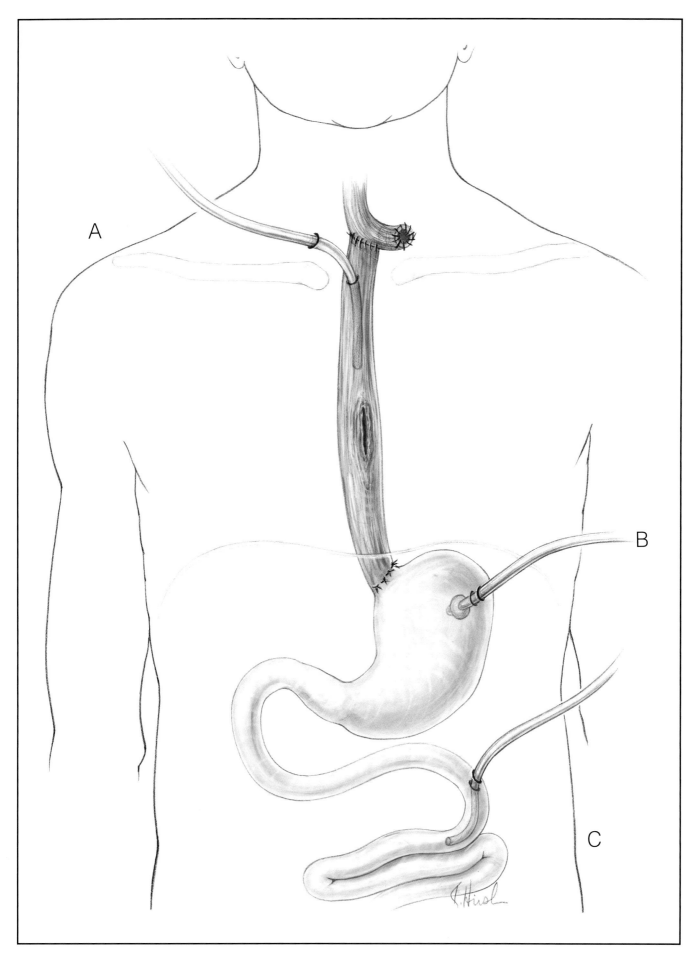

# *Index*

*Page numbers followed by f represent figures.*

## *A*

Achalasia, 156–159
  esophagomyotomy and partial fundoplication for, 156, 157f
  treatment of, 156
Adenocarcinoma
  distal esophagectomy for, 96, 97f
  of distal intra-abdominal segment of esophagus, esophagectomy without thoracotomy for, 42–51
  reconstruction after removal of, 30
  total gastrectomy for, 96, 97f
Anastomosis
  after palliative esophagectomy, 40, 41f
  after right thoracotomy, 34
  colocolic, in esophageal reconstruction with isoperistaltic left colon, 68, 69f
  cologastric, in substernal left colon bypass, 104, 105f
  end-to-end, in substernal left colon bypass, 106, 107f
  in esophageal diversion, 180, 181f
  in esophageal reconstruction with isoperistaltic left colon, 68
  in esophageal reconstruction with whole stomach, 58, 59f, 60, 61f
  esophagocolic, in esophageal reconstruction with isoperistaltic left colon, 70, 71f
  esophagogastric, 94, 95f
  esophagojejunal, through left thoracotomy, 86, 87f, 88, 89f
  leakage rates for, 76
  in long segment interposition, 74, 75f
  of proximal and distal jejunum, 82, 83f
  stapled, advantages and disadvantages of, 76
  in subcutaneous right colon bypass, 112, 113f
  techniques for, 76, 77f
    continuous suture, 78, 79f
Antireflux repairs
  Collis gastroplasty and, 142–147
  Mark IV
    for achalasia, 158, 159f
    for diffuse esophageal spasm, 160, 161f
  Thal patch and, 148, 149f
  transabdominal, 128–131
    completion of, 130, 131f
    gastroesophageal junction mobilization in, 128, 129f
    suture placement in, 128, 129f, 130, 131f
  transthoracic, 116–123
    Belsey Mark IV reconstruction in, 120, 121f, 122, 123f

    cross-section of, 122, 123f
    distal esophagus repositioning in, 118, 119f
    gastroesophageal junction mobilization in, 120, 121f
    opening of greater peritoneal cavity in, 118, 119f
    peritoneal cavity entry, 116, 117f
    stomach delivery in, 118, 119f
    transthoracic Nissen fundoplication, 124–127
Aorta, 16, 17f, 21f, 27f
  exposure of, 44, 45f
Arcuate ligament, identification of, in Hill posterior gastropexy, 132, 133f
Artery(ies)
  Belsey's, 119f
  celiac, dissection of, 26
  esophageal, avulsed, 49f
  gastric, 40, 41f
    division of, in substernal colon bypass, 108, 109f
  gastroepiploic, 63f
  inferior phrenic, 26, 27f
  innominate, 16, 17f
  intercostal, 35f
  left gastric, 26, 27f
  left gastroepiploic, division of, 54
  midcolic, division of, in long segment interposition, 72
  omental, 40, 41f
  phrenic, 119f
  right gastroepiploic, as blood supply in esophageal reconstruction, 54
  right intercostal, ligation of, 32, 33f
  splenic, 26, 27f
  Sweet's, ligation and division of, 22
Azygos vein, 10, 11f, 21f, 26, 27f, 35f, 37f, 45f
  ligation of, 44, 45f

## *B*

Balfour retractor, 4, 8, 10, 22
Barrett's esophagus, 72
  reconstruction after removal of, 30
Barrett's ulcer, esophageal rupture caused by, 175
Belsey Mark IV reconstruction, 120, 121f, 122, 123f
Belsey operation, 115
Belsey's artery, 119f
Bradycardia, risk of, 46
Bypass procedures, 99–113
  subcutaneous right colon, 110–113
  substernal left colon, 100–107
  substernal stomach, 108, 109f

# C

Carcinoma. *See also* Neoplasms, malignant
   from proximal stomach to distal esophagus,
      gastrectomy for, 92–95
Cardia, calibration of, in Hill posterior gastropexy,
   134, 135f
Celiac artery, dissection of, 26
Cervical esophagus, approaches to, 12, 13f, 14, 15f
Collis gastroplasty, 142–147
   gastric vessel division in, 142, 143f
   indications for, 142
   Nissen fundoplication or partial Mark IV repair
      in, 146, 147f
   suture placement in, 144, 145f
   swallowing tube elongation in, 144, 145f
   through left thoracotomy, 142, 143f
   total fundoplication around gastric tube in, 146,
      147f
Colon
   isoperistaltic left
      blood supply of, 62
      in esophageal reconstruction, 62–71
      reconstruction after total gastrectomy, 96, 97f
      reconstructive advantages of, 62
   transverse, transection point for, 64, 65f
Colon bypass, substernal. *See* Substernal left colon
      bypass
Connell suture, 78
Continuous suture anastomotic technique, 78, 79f
Coronary vein, 26, 27f, 45f
   ligation of, 44, 45f

# D

Deaver retractor, 4
Diaphragm
   excision with electrocautery, 42
   incision of, 24, 25f
   retraction of, 28, 29f
Digestion, restoring partial capacity for, 94
Diverticula
   epiphrenic. *See* Epiphrenic diverticulum
   Zenker's, 162–165

# E

Electrocautery, in esophagectomy without
      thoracotomy, 42
Endothoracic fascia, 39f, 117f
Epiphrenic diverticulum, 166–171
   esophageal mobilization in, 166, 167f
   left thoracotomy for, 166, 167f
   myotomy in, 170, 171f
   resection of, 168, 169f
   suture placement in, 168, 169f
Esophageal artery, avulsed, 49f
Esophageal diversion, 180, 181f
   feeding jejunostomy in, 180, 181f
   laparotomy in, 180, 181f
Esophagectomy
   avoidance of, in infected esophageal rupture, 180
   distal, 92
      for adenocarcinoma, 96, 97f
   en bloc
      completion of, 30, 31f
      through left thoracotomy, 20–31
      through right thoracotomy, 32–35
   palliative, 19

   anastomosis after, 40, 41f
      through right thoracotomy, 36–41
   through right thoracotomy, closed chest, before
      substernal left colon bypass, 100, 101f
   without reconstruction, bypass procedures for, 99
   without thoracotomy, 19, 42–51
      reconstruction with whole stomach after, 54–61
Esophagitis
   avoiding risk of, 50
   reflux, strictures in, 141. *See also* Strictures
Esophagomyotomy, for achalasia, 156–159
Esophagus
   benign stenosis of, jejunal interposition technique
      for, 80–89
   diffuse spasm of, 160, 161f
   division of, at sternal manubrium level, 180, 181f
   maneuvers for freeing from pulmonary hila,
      aortic arch, and tracheal bifurcation
      region, 48, 49f
   midportion of, tumors of, 36
   operative approaches to, 1–17
      abdominal, 2, 3f
      cervical, 12, 13f, 14, 15f
      cervical with partial sternotomy, 16, 17f
      thoracic, 6–9. *See also* Thoracotomy
   reconstruction of, 53–97
      by gastric tube interposition, 90, 91f
      with isoperistaltic left colon, 62–71
      by jejunal interposition, 80–89
      with long segment interposition, 72–75
      with whole stomach, 54–61
   rupture of, 175–181
      causes of, 175
      esophageal diversion for, 180, 181f
      pleural patch for repair of, 176–179
      primary repair of, 178
   thoracic, total removal of, 20. *See also*
      Esophagectomy, en bloc
   Zenker's diverticulum of, 162–165
External oblique muscle, 2, 3f

# F

Falciforme ligament, division of, 2, 3f
Fascia, endothoracic, 39f, 117f
Feeding jejunostomy, in esophageal diversion, 180,
   181f
Fundoplication
   Guarner partial, 138, 139f
   intrathoracic total. *See* Intrathoracic total
      fundoplication
   Nissen transthoracic. *See* Transthoracic Nissen
      fundoplication
   partial, for achalasia, 156–159

# G

Gastrectomy, total
   with adenocarcinoma of cardia, 96
   reconstruction after, 92–97
Gastric arteries, 40, 41f
   left, 26, 27f
Gastric fundus, reattachment of, 70, 71f
Gastric tube interposition, 90, 91f
   disadvantages of, 90
Gastroepiploic artery, 63f
Gastrohepatic ligament, 42, 43f
Gastropexy, Hill posterior. *See* Hill posterior
      gastropexy

Gastroplasty, Collis. *See* Collis gastroplasty
Gelfoam, use in esophageal reconstruction with
    isoperistaltic left colon, 68
Guarner operation, 115. *See also* Antireflux repairs,
    transabdominal
Guarner partial fundoplication, 138, 139f

## H

Hepatic flexure, 64, 65f
Hernia, hiatal, iatrogenic, in intrathoracic total
    fundoplication, 152
Hiatus
    abdominal approaches to, 2, 3f
    enlargement of, in intrathoracic total
        fundoplication, 150, 151f
    exposure of, 4, 5f
Hill operation, 115. *See also* Antireflux repairs,
    transabdominal
Hill posterior gastropexy, 132–137
    arcuate ligament identification in, 132, 133f
    cardia calibration in, 134, 135f
    cardia retraction in, 132, 133f
    final pressure recording in, 136
    initiation of, 134, 135f
Hypotension, risk of, 46

## I

Incisions
    abdominal, 2, 3f
    of diaphragm, 24, 25f
    left thoracotomy, 6–9
    pericardial, 28, 29f
    right cervical, 46
    right subcostal, 2, 3f, 42, 43f
    for right thoracotomy, 10, 32, 33f
    sternal, 16, 17f
    thoracoabdominal, 6, 7f
    transverse collar, 12, 13f
Innominate artery, 16, 17f
Innominate vein, 16
Intercostal artery, 35f
Intercostal muscles, division of, 6, 7f
Intercostal vein, 35f
Internal oblique muscle, 2, 3f
Intrathoracic total fundoplication, 150–153
    anchoring of, 152, 153f
    diaphragm cuff excision in, 150, 151f
    hiatal enlargement in, 150, 151f
    indication for, 150
    thoracotomy for, 150, 151f

## J

Jejunal interposition technique, 80–89
    indications for, 80
Jejunal loop
    reconstruction after total gastrectomy, 92–95
    roux-en-y, 108
Jejunostomy, feeding, in esophageal diversion, 180,
    181f

## L

Lambert stitch, 78
Laparotomy, in esophageal diversion, 180, 181f
Latissimus dorsi muscle, 6, 7f
Leiomyoma, 172, 173f

determining operative approach to, 172
    symptoms of, 172
Lesser omentum, 119f
Ligaments
    falciforme, division of, 2, 3f
    gastrohepatic, 42, 43f
    pulmonary, 33f
        division of, 8, 9f, 10, 11f, 22
    of Treitz, 92, 93f
    triangular, 4, 5f
Lye strictures, bypass procedures for, 99
Lymph node, subcarinal, 23f

## M

Mark IV repair
    for achalasia, 158, 159f
    in Collis gastroplasty, 146, 147f
    for diffuse esophageal spasm, 160, 161f
Mediastinum, exposure of, 8, 9f, 28, 29f
Microcirculation, Gelfoam for avoiding damage
    to, 68
Motor disorders, 155–173. *See also* specific disorders
Muscle(s)
    abdominal, 2, 3f
    latissimus dorsi, 6, 7f
    omohyoid, 12, 13f
    paraspinal, 6, 7f
    serratus, division of, 22
    serratus anterior, 6, 7f
    sternocleidomastoid, 12, 13f
    sternohyoid, 12, 13f
    sternothyroid, 12, 13f
    thyrohyoid, 12, 13f
Myotomy
    for achalasia, 156, 157f
    for diffuse esophageal spasm, 160, 161f
    for epiphrenic diverticulum, 168, 169f
    for Zenker's diverticulum, 164, 165f

## N

Neoplasms
    of cervical esophagus, 16
    esophageal rupture caused by, 175
    malignant, resection for, 19–51
    of midportion of esophagus, 36
    preoperative staging of, 19
    of thoracic inlet, 16
Nerves, vagus, 121f
Nissen fundoplication
    in Collis gastroplasty, 146, 147f
    transthoracic. *See* Transthoracic Nissen
        fundoplication
Nissen operation, 115

## O

Omental arteries, 40, 41f
Omentum
    elevation of, 24, 25f
    embryology of, 24
    lesser, 119f
Omohyoid muscle, 12, 13f

## P

Paraspinal muscle, 6, 7f
Pericardium, 11f, 21f, 33f, 35f

Peritoneum, 39f, 117f
Pharynx, Zenker's diverticulum of, 162–165
Phrenic artery, 119f
Phrenoesophageal membrane, 117f, 119f
    resection of, 38, 39f
Pleura, 35f
Pleural patch
    esophageal exposure for, 176, 177f
    for esophageal rupture, 176–179
    indications for, 178
Pulmonary ligament, 33f
    division of, 8, 9f, 10, 11f, 22
Pulmonary veins, 11f
Pyloromyotomy, 50, 54, 55f
    closure of, 56, 57f
    in esophageal reconstruction with whole stomach,
        60
    in substernal colon bypass, 108
Pyloroplasty
    in esophageal reconstruction with whole stomach,
        60
    long, 54
    in substernal colon bypass, 108

# R

Rectus abdominus muscle, 2, 3f
Reflux
    control of, 115. *See also* Antireflux repairs
    strictures induced by. *See* Strictures
Retractors
    Balfour, 8, 10, 22
    Balfour self-retaining, 4
    Deaver, 4
    Tuffier, 16
    "upper hand," 4
Roux-en-y jejunal loop, 108

# S

Serratus anterior muscle, 6, 7
Serratus muscle, division of, 22
Spasm, diffuse esophageal, 160, 161f
Splenic artery, 26, 27f
Splenic flexure, 64, 65f
Squamous cell carcinoma, reconstruction after
    removal of, 30
Sternocleidomastoid muscle, 12, 13f
Sternothyroid muscle, 12, 13f
Sternotomy, partial, with cervical approach to
    esophagus, 16, 17f
Stomach
    mobilization through hiatus, 40
    torsion of, avoiding, 58, 59f
Stomach bypass, substernal. *See* Substernal stomach
    bypass
Strictures, 141–153
    Collis gastroplasty for repair of, 142–147
    intrathoracic total fundoplication for,150–153
    Thal patch for repair of, 148, 149f
Subcutaneous right colon bypass procedure,
    110–113
    anastomosis in, 112, 113f
    division of transverse colon, mesocolon, ileum,

    and mesentery in, 110, 111f
    incisions for, 110, 111f
    tunnel creation in, 110, 111f
Substernal left colon bypass
    end-to-end anastomosis in, 106, 107f
    indications for, 108
Substernal left colon bypass procedure
    cologastric anastomosis in, 104, 105f
    esophagectomy through right thoracotomy,
        closed chest preceding, 100, 101f
    incision for, 100, 101f
    transverse cervical incision in, 102, 103f
    tunnel creation in, 102, 103f
Sweet's artery, ligation and division of, 22

# T

Thal patch, 148, 149f
    fundoplication in, 148, 149f
    partial-thickness skin graft in, 148, 149f
    thoracotomy for, 148, 149f
Thoracic duct, 21f, 27f, 35f, 45f
Thoracic inlet, neoplasms of, 16
Thoracotomy
    esophagectomy without, 19
    left, 6–9
        en bloc esophagectomy through, 32–35
        opening of, 8, 9f
    right, 10, 11f
        indications for, 10
        reconstruction after, 34
        standard or palliative esophagectomy through,
            36–41
Thorax, cross-section of, 20, 21f
    left, en bloc esophagectomy through, 20–31
Thyrohyoid muscle, 12, 13f
Tracheoesophageal fistula, bypass procedures for, 99
Transthoracic Nissen fundoplication, 124–127
    completion of, 124, 125f
    fundus manipulation following, 126, 127f
    suture placement in, 124, 125f
Treitz, ligament of, 92, 93f
Triangular ligament, 4, 5f
Tuffier retractor, 16
Tumors. *See* Neoplasms, malignant

# V

Vagus nerves, 121f
Veins
    azygos, 10, 11f, 21f, 26, 27f, 35f, 37f, 45f
        ligation of, 44, 45f
    coronary, 26, 27f, 45f
        ligation of, 44, 45f
    innominate, 16
    intercostal, 33f, 35f
    midthyroid, 14, 15f
    pulmonary, 11f
    right intercostal, ligation of, 32, 33f

# Z

Zenker's diverticulum, 162–165
    myotomy for, 164, 165f